Hematopoietic Stem Cell Transplantation for Immunodeficiency, Part I

Guest Editor

CHAIM M. ROIFMAN, MD, FRCPC, FCACB

IMMUNOLOGY AND ALLERGY CLINICS OF NORTH AMERICA

www.immunology.theclinics.com

Consulting Editor
RAFEUL ALAM, MD, PhD

February 2010 • Volume 30 • Number 1

SAUNDERS an imprint of ELSEVIER, Inc.

W.B. SAUNDERS COMPANY
A Division of Elsevier Inc.

1600 John F. Kennedy Blvd., ● Suite 1800 ● Philadelphia, PA 19103-2899.

http://www.theclinics.com

IMMUNOLOGY AND ALLERGY CLINICS OF NORTH AMERICA Volume 30, Number 1
February 2010 ISSN 0889–8561, ISBN-13: 978-1-4377-1828-7

Editor: Patrick Manley

Immunology and Allergy Clinics of North America (ISSN 0889–8561) is published quarterly by Elsevier Inc., 360 Park Avenue South, New York, NY 10010-1710. Months of issue are February, May, August, and November. Periodicals postage paid at New York, NY and additional mailing offices. Subscription prices are $254.00 per year for US individuals, $373.00 per year for US institutions, $123.00 per year for US students and residents, $312.00 per year for Canadian individuals, $178.00 per year for Canadian students, $463.00 per year for Canadian institutions, $354.00 per year for international individuals, $463.00 per year for international institutions, $178.00 per year for international students. To receive student/resident rate, orders must be accompanied by name of affiliated institution, date of term, and the *signature* of program/residency coordinator on institution letterhead. Orders will be billed at individual rate until proof of status is received. Foreign air speed delivery is included in all *Clinics* subscription prices. All prices are subject to change without notice. **POSTMASTER**: Send address changes to *Immunology and Allergy Clinics of North America,* Elsevier Health Sciences Division Subscription Customer Service, 3251 Riverport Lane, Maryland Heights, MO 63043. **Customer Service: 1-800-654-2452 (US and Canada); 314-447-8871 (outside U.S. and Canada). Fax: 314-447-8029. E-mail: journalscustomerservice-usa@elsevier.com (for print support); journalsonlinesupport-usa@elsevier. com (for online support).**

Reprints. For copies of 100 or more, of articles in this publication, please contact the Commercial Reprints Department, Elsevier Inc., 360 Park Avenue South, New York, New York 10010-1710. Tel. (212) 633-3812, Fax: (212) 462-1935, E-mail: reprints@elsevier.com.

Immunology and Allergy Clinics of North America is covered in MEDLINE/PubMed (Index Medicus), Current Contents/Life Sciences, Science Citation Index, ISI/BIOMED, Chemical Abstracts, and EMBASE/Excerpta Medica.

Printed and bound by CPI Group (UK) Ltd, Croydon, CR0 4YY

Transferred to Digital Print 2011

Contributors

CONSULTING EDITOR

RAFEUL ALAM, MD, PhD
Veda and Chauncey Ritter Chair in Immunology, Professor, and Director, Division
of Immunology and Allergy, National Jewish Health; and University of Colorado Health
Sciences Center, Denver, Colorado

GUEST EDITOR

CHAIM M. ROIFMAN, MD, FRCPC, FCACB
Donald and Audrey Campbell Chair of Immunology; Professor of Pediatrics and
Immunology, University of Toronto; Director, Canadian Center for Primary
Immunodeficiency; Head, Division of Immunology and Allergy, Department of Pediatrics,
The Hospital for Sick Children, Toronto, Ontario, Canada

AUTHORS

SUNG W. CHOI, MD
Assistant Professor, Department of Pediatrics, Blood and Marrow Transplant Program,
University of Michigan Medical School, Ann Arbor, Michigan

MORTON J. COWAN, MD
Professor and Chief, Division of Pediatric Blood and Marrow Transplantation, University
of California, San Francisco, San Francisco, California

M. TERESA DE LA MORENA, MD
Associate Professor of Pediatrics and Internal Medicine, Division of Allergy and
Immunology, University of Texas Southwestern Medical Center in Dallas, Dallas, Texas

CHRISTOPHER C. DVORAK, MD
Assistant Professor, Division of Pediatric Blood and Marrow Transplantation, University
of California, San Francisco, San Francisco, California

JAMES L.M. FERRARA, MD, DSc
Director, Blood and Marrow Transplant Program, Ruth Heyn Professor of Pediatric
Oncology, American Cancer Society Clinical Research Professor, Department of Internal
Medicine and Pediatrics, University of Michigan Medical School, Ann Arbor, Michigan

WILHELM FRIEDRICH, MD
Associate Professor, Department of Pediatrics, University of Ulm, Ulm, Germany

RICHARD A. GATTI, MD
Distinguished Professor, Department of Pathology and Laboratory Medicine, Macdonald
Research Laboratories, University of California, Los Angeles School of Medicine,
Los Angeles, California

EYAL GRUNEBAUM, MD
Associate Professor Pediatrics, Division of Clinical Immunology and Allergy, Department of Pediatrics, The Hospital for Sick Children, University of Toronto, Toronto, Ontario, Canada

DAVID HAGIN, MD
Department of Immunology, Weizmann Institute of Science, Rehovot, Israel

MANFRED HÖNIG, MD
Department of Pediatrics, University of Ulm, Ulm, Germany

NEENA KAPOOR, MD
Professor of Pediatrics, Department of Pediatrics, University of Southern California Keck School of Medicine; Clinical Director, Bone Marrow Transplantation Program, Division of Research Immunology/Bone Marrow Transplantation, Childrens Hospital Los Angeles, Los Angeles, California

DONALD B. KOHN, MD
Professor of Microbiology, Immunology and Molecular Genetics; and Professor of Pediatrics, University of California, Los Angeles, Los Angeles, California

JOHN E. LEVINE, MD
Professor, Clinical Director of Pediatric Blood and Marrow Transplant Program, Department of Internal Medicine and Pediatrics, University of Michigan Medical School, Ann Arbor, Michigan

RICHARD J. O'REILLY, MD
Chair, Department of Pediatrics; Chief, Pediatric Bone Marrow Transplant Service; Claire L. Tow Chair in Pediatric Oncology Research, Memorial Sloan Kettering Cancer Center, New York, New York

ROBERTSON PARKMAN, MD
Professor of Pediatrics, Division of Research Immunology/BMT, and The Saban Research Institute, Childrens Hospital Los Angeles; Department of Pediatrics, Molecular Microbiology and Immunology, University of Southern California Keck School of Medicine, Los Angeles, California

JOEL M. RAPPEPORT, MD
Department of Internal Medicine, Yale University School of Medicine, New Haven, Connecticut

YAIR REISNER, PhD
Chairman, Department of Immunology, Weizmann Institute of Science, Rehovot, Israel

CHAIM M. ROIFMAN, MD, FRCPC, FCACB
Donald and Audrey Campbell Chair of Immunology; Professor of Pediatrics and Immunology, University of Toronto; Director, Canadian Center for Primary Immunodeficiency; Head, Division of Immunology and Allergy, Department of Pediatrics, The Hospital for Sick Children, Toronto, Ontario, Canada

AMI J. SHAH, MD
Associate Professor of Clinical Pediatrics, Division of Research Immunology/Bone
Marrow Transplantation, Department of Pediatrics, The Saban Research Institute,
Childrens Hospital Los Angeles, University of Southern California Keck School of
Medicine, Los Angeles, California

PAUL VEYS, MBBS, FRCP, FRCPath, FRCPCH
Director of Blood and Marrow Transplantation, Department of BMT, Great Ormond Street
Hospital for Children NHS Trust; Reader in Stem Cell Transplantation, Molecular
Immunology Unit, University College London Institute of Child Health, London,
United Kingdom

Contents

The last 40 years has seen the emergence of hematopoietic stem cell transplantation as a therapeutic modality for fatal diseases and as a curative option for individuals born with inherited disorders that carry limited life expectancy and poor quality of life. Despite the rarity of many primary immunodeficiency diseases, these disorders have led the way toward innovative therapies and further provide insights into mechanisms of immunologic reconstitution applicable to all hematopoietic stem cell transplants. This article represents a historical perspective of the early investigators and their contributions. It also reviews the parallel work that oncologists and immunologists have undertaken to treat both primary immunodeficiencies and hematologic malignancies.

It is now more than 40 years since the first successful allogeneic hematopoietic stem cell transplantation (HSCT) for a child with severe combined immunodeficiency (SCID). In the succeeding years, HSCT for SCID patients have represented only a small portion of the total number of allogeneic HSCT performed. Nevertheless, the clinical and biologic importance of the patients transplanted for SCID has continued. SCID patients were the first to be successfully transplanted with nonsibling related bone marrow, unrelated bone marrow, T-cell depleted HSCT, and genetically corrected (gene transfer) autologous HSC. Many of the biologic insights now widely applied to allogeneic HSCT were first identified in the transplantation of SCID patients. This article reviews the clinical and biologic lessons that have been learned from HSCT for SCID patients, and how the information has impacted the general field of allogeneic HSCT.

Curative treatment of Severe Combined Immunodeficiency (SCID) by Hematopoietic Cell Transplantation (HCT) remains a challenge, in particular in infants presenting with serious, poorly controllable complications. In the absence of a matched family donor, HLA-haploidentical transplantation from parental donors represents a uniformly and readily available treatment option, offering a high chance to be successful. Concerning outcomes of HCT in SCID, other important parameters beside survival need to be taken into consideration, in particular the stability and robustness of the graft and its function, as well as potential late complications, related either to the disease or to the treatment.

Since the early 1980s T-cell depletion has allowed haploidentical bone marrow transplantation to be performed in patients with primary immunodeficiency for whom a matched sibling donor was not available, without causing severe graft versus host disease (GVHD). This review article presents the available data in the literature on survival, GVHD, and immune reconstitution in different categories of patients, with special emphasis on the impact of different T-cell depletion methods.

Severe combined immunodeficiency (SCID) is fatal in infancy unless corrected with allogeneic bone marrow transplants (BMT), preferably from a family-related genotypically HLA-identical donor (RID) or phenotypically HLA-matched family donor (PMD). For the majority of SCID patients, such donors are not available; Therefore, parents who are HLA-haploidentical donors (HID) or HLA-matched unrelated donors (MUD) have been used. MUD BMT are associated with increased frequency of acute graft versus host disease, which can be controlled by high doses of steroids. HID BMT are associated with increased frequency of short- and long-term graft failure, need for repeated transplants, fatal pneumonitis, impaired immune reconstitution, and long-term complications, contributing to lower survival. In conclusion, the excellent long-term survival, immune reconstitution, and normal quality of life after MUD BMT suggests that in the absence of RID or PMD, MUD BMT should be offered for patients suffering from SCID.

Allogeneic hematopoietic cell transplantation (HCT) is an important therapeutic option for various malignant and nonmalignant conditions. As allogeneic HCT continues to increase, greater attention is given to improvements in supportive care, infectious prophylaxis, immunosuppressive medications, and DNA-based tissue typing. However, graft versus host disease (GVHD) remains the most frequent and serious complication following allogeneic HCT and limits the broader application of this important therapy. Recent advances in the understanding of the pathogenesis of GVHD have led to new approaches to its management, including using it to preserve the graft versus leukemia effect following allogeneic transplant.

This article reviews the important elements in the complex immunologic interactions involving cytokine networks, chemokine gradients, and the direct mediators of cellular cytotoxicity that cause clinical GVHD, and discusses the risk factors and strategies for management of GVHD.

Many advances have been made since the first successful hematopoietic cell transplants (HCT) in children with primary immunodeficiency disorders (PID) were reported 40 years ago, and many children with PID can now be cured from their otherwise lethal disorders through well-matched HCT procedures. Preexisting morbidity and infection remain the principal adverse factors for poor outcomes with HCT. To improve current results, earlier diagnosis, well-tolerated pretransplant conditioning regimens, and promotion of immune reconstitution need to be considered. This article addresses modifications in the conditioning regimen that might lead to further improvement in HCT outcomes.

Inherited defects in components of the nonhomologous end-joining DNA repair mechanism produce a T–B–NK+ severe combined immunodeficiency disease (SCID) characterized by heightened sensitivity to ionizing radiation. Patients with the radiosensitive form of SCID may also have increased short- and long-term sensitivity to the alkylator-based chemotherapy regimens that are traditionally used for conditioning before allogeneic hematopoietic cell transplantation (HCT). Known causes of radiosensitive SCID include deficiencies of Artemis, DNA ligase IV, DNA-dependent protein kinase catalytic subunit, and Cernunnos-XLF, all of which have been treated with HCT. Because of these patients' sensitivity to certain forms of chemotherapy, the approach to donor selection and the type of conditioning regimen used for a patient with radiosensitive SCID requires careful consideration. Significantly more research needs to be done to determine the long-term outcomes of patients with radiosensitive SCID after HCT and to discover novel nontoxic approaches to HCT that might benefit those patients with intrinsic radiosensitivity and chemosensitivity as well as potentially all patients undergoing an HCT.

Hematopoietic stem cell transplantation (HSCT) has offered a curative approach for treating patients with severe combined immunodeficiency (SCID). However, HSCT may have long-term effects on some of these patients. This article reviews the literature regarding long-term neurocognitive function of patients who have received HSCT for SCID, including the effect of disease-specific characteristics, psychosocial factors, being a chronically ill child, and transplant-related factors.

THE CLINICS ARE NOW AVAILABLE ONLINE!

Access your subscription at:
www.theclinics.com

Foreword
Hematopoietic Stem Cell Transplantation for Primary Immunodeficiency Disorders

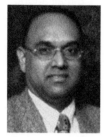

Rafeul Alam, MD, PhD
Consulting Editor

Since the discovery of the blood group in 1901 by Nobel laureate Karl Landsteiner and the first successful bone marrow transplantation in 1956 by another Nobel laureate, Donnall Thomas, we have come a long way to understanding the fundamental principles of transplantation immunology and clinical transplantation. Hematopoietic stem cell transplantation in primary immunodeficiency disorders, especially in severe combined immunodeficiency (SCID), has been a prime example of progress that this discipline has made and the difficulties it faces. The use of haplocompatible related donors has reduced the length of time required to perform transplantation and has improved the outcome. Similarly, the availability of cord blood stem cells has opened new opportunities. The requirement for preconditioning before transplantation remains an open question. Early diagnosis and transplantation remain challenges. In this regard, newborn screening for interleukin-7 and T cell receptor excision circles may become an extremely useful tool. Diagnosing SCID and performing transplantation in utero is an exciting new approach that will certainly be further explored. Lessons learned from hematopoietic stem cell transplantation in primary immunodeficiency disorders will be enormously valuable in this era of gene therapy. Dr Chaim Roifman, a leader in the field, has invited a group of experts to update us on the progress in stem cell transplantation in SCID and to describe the challenges it faces. Topics in this issue include a history of bone marrow transplantation, SCID, hematopoietic

Supported by National Institutes of Health grants RO1 AI059719 and AI68088, PPG HL 36577, and N01 HHSN272200700048C.

Immunol Allergy Clin N Am 30 (2010) xi–xii
doi:10.1016/j.iac.2009.12.001   immunology.theclinics.com

stem cell transplantation in SCID, sources of stem cells for transplantation, and graft-versus-host disease.

Rafeul Alam, MD, PhD
Division of Allergy & Immunology
National Jewish Health & University of Colorado
Denver Health Sciences Center
1400 Jackson Street, Denver, CO 80206, USA

E-mail address:
alamr@njc.org

Preface

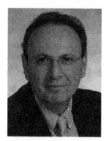

Chaim M. Roifman, MD, FRCPC, FCACB
Guest Editor

Stem cell transplantation has been a life-saving procedure for patients with primary immunodeficiency for more than 4 decades. Using a family-related HLA-identical donor (RID) has been so successful (with 90% survival) that it meets consensus as first choice of therapy when stem cell therapy is recommended for primary immunodeficiency. Unfortunately, RID is available in fewer than 20% of cases. Even when available, it remains an imperfect procedure, being rarely associated with complications, such as graft-versus-host disease (GVHD). Opinions defer whether patients receiving RID should be given GVHD prophylaxis. Another controversy involves the use of conditioning, especially in cases with significant residual T cell numbers and function. Critical assessment of these practices is sorely needed.

In the absence of RID, stem cells from mismatched related donors, usually a parent, were traditionally used. Wide use of this modality of treatment was triggered by Yair Raisner's pioneer work regarding the use of lectins for T cell depletion. While this and other T cell depletion procedures saved many lives, it definitely did not live up to its promise of replacing RID. Engraftment using this method has been partial at best, necessitating multiple repeated transplants. Moreover, long-term immune reconstitution may not be achieved as some cases show a late loss of graft, a decade or more posttransplantation. Moreover, survival rate using haploidentical donors has been consistently hovering around 50% or less according to most large studies. Mortality is caused by severe infections, pulmonary complications, or GVHD.

The growing number of bone marrow registries worldwide made the use of an unrelated match donor (MUD) possible. The use of MUDs was a major turning point in the field of immune reconstitution for primary immunodeficiency disease. From small case studies to large trials, survival rates were consistently better than 70% to 75% with no exceptions. Hemopoietic reconstitution is rapid and so is immune recovery, reducing substantially the frequency of life-threatening infections. Moreover, long-term immune reconstitution is universally robust. Unfortunately, GVHD remains a major complication of this mode of treatment, despite routine use of GVHD prophylaxis.

Another, true or perceived problem is the use of myeloablative conditioning before MUD or mismatched related donor transplants. Although others and we have shown

Immunol Allergy Clin N Am 30 (2010) xiii–xiv
doi:10.1016/j.iac.2009.12.002   immunology.theclinics.com

the obvious benefits of conditioning, concerns remain about the possible toxicity of myeloablative regimens, especially with the use of busulfan and cyclophosphamide. This prompted the move to modify conditioning using reduced-intensity regimens. Such attempts should be encouraged, provided they are carefully and prospectively studied. However, so far there hasn't been sufficient evidence for an effective and safe alternative to busulfan/cyclophosphamide. To date, it remains unclear whether engraftment is complete or sustained after reduced-intensity regimens and the short- and long-term toxicity of drugs replacing cyclophosphamide or busulfan have not been critically assessed in this setting.

This issue provides a review of many important aspects of stem cell therapy for primary immunodeficiency. Experts in the field present here the most up-to-date experience in various methods of stem cell manipulation and transplantations as well as the latest information about complications associated with this procedure and their management.

DEDICATION

This issue is dedicated to Robert A. Good, father of modern clinical immunology and cellular engineering, and world-renowned pioneer in investigations of host defenses through the study of the molecular basis of inherited immune deficiency and its treatment.

Chaim M. Roifman, MD, FRCPC, FCACB
Division of Immunology and Allergy
Department of Pediatrics
The Hospital for Sick Children
555 University Avenue
Toronto, Ontario M5G 1X8
Canada

E-mail address:
croifman@sickkids.ca

A History of Bone Marrow Transplantation

M. Teresa de la Morena, MD[a],*, Richard A. Gatti, MD[b]

KEYWORDS

- Bone marrow transplantation • History
- Primary immunodeficiency diseases

Five decades ago, the concept of bone marrow transplantation to treat humans with inherited diseases of immune function, marrow failure syndromes, and leukemia was met with much skepticism, degrees of enthusiasm, and many disappointments. Transferring what was known from experimental animal models to humans was met with many challenges, and such beginnings were very difficult. Certain death due to the primary disease, characterized the outcomes of individuals who were considered for transplantation. Consequently these patients became the sickest on the medical wards, and the physicians caring for such patients were posed with many questions regarding the benefits of such attempts. One of the major obstacles, graft-versus-host disease (GVHD) was "incomparably more violent than in (inbred) rodents" as stated by Bekkum and van de Vries.[1] Yet through the recognition and subsequent understanding of fundamental immunologic processes, medical resiliency, and the stubborn determination of a few pioneers, bone marrow transplantation changed from an insurmountable therapeutic option for a limited number of patients to a form of therapy for 30,000 to 50,000 people worldwide annually.[2] Hematopoietic stem cell transplantation (HSCT) today is no longer a treatment modality for lethal diseases such as primary immunodeficiency diseases (PIDs) or malignancies but a valid approach of "cellular engineering"[3] for solid tumors, hemoglobinopathies, autoimmune diseases, inherited disorders of metabolism, histiocytic disorders, and other nonmalignancies.[2]

[a] Department of Pediatrics and Internal Medicine, Division of Allergy and Immunology, University of Texas Southwestern Medical Center in Dallas, 5323 Harry Hines Boulevard, Dallas, TX 75390-9063, USA
[b] Department of Pathology and Laboratory Medicine, 675 Charles Young Drive South, Room 4-736, Macdonald Research Laboratories, University of California Los Angeles School of Medicine, Los Angeles, CA 90095-1732, USA
* Corresponding author.
E-mail address: maite.delamorena@utsouthwestern.edu (M.T. de la Morena).

Immunol Allergy Clin N Am 30 (2010) 1–15
doi:10.1016/j.iac.2009.11.005
0889-8561/10/$ – see front matter © 2010 Elsevier Inc. All rights reserved.

This article represents a historical perspective of the early investigators and their contributions. It also reviews the parallel work that oncologists and immunologists have undertaken to treat both PIDs and hematologic malignancies.

THE EARLY DAYS

The idea of removing damaged parts of the body and replacing them with healthy organs has been an aim shared by physicians since ancient times. An early discussion on the use of bone marrow was outline in 1896 by Quine in the Chairman's address of the Journal of the American Medical Association, where he discussed the "remedial application of bone marrow extracts."[4] However, the physical consequences of World War II brought research in tissue transplantation to the forefront: skin grafts were needed for burn victims; blood transfusions required careful ABO blood typing and monitoring of blood group antibodies; and high doses of radiation lead to marrow failure and death, with little understanding of radiobiological mechanisms.

By the early 1940s, it was clear that phagocytes were macrophages, antibodies were part of the gamma-globulin fraction of serum proteins (as defined by their electrophoretic mobility),[5] and the "small lymphocytes" were influenced by adrenal hormones.[6] At the request of the Medical Research Council during World War II, Medawar[7] started work on the study of rejection of skin grafts, a priority for the treatment of burn victims. Early versions of immunologic tolerance and alloreactivity were published. In 1945, Ray Owen in Wisconsin, while studying the inheritance of blood group antigens in freemartin cattle, described how fraternal twin cattle were chimeric for 2 blood groups, their own and that of the twin.[8] At the turn of the century, Loeb[9] had been unable to transfer tumors from Japanese waltzing mice to different strains of mice, whereas such tumors grew easily within the inbred strain. To Gorer[10] and subsequently to Snell,[11–13] we owe the identification of the major histocompatibility complex (MHC) genes in rodents (H-2 system in the mouse).

Medawar assimilated this background and provided convincing evidence that graft rejection was an immunologic phenomenon[7] linked to histocompatibility antigens. Subsequently with Billingham and Brent, he designed a series of hallmark experiments, in which he demonstrated the induction of immunologic tolerance.[14] Yet within the first few lines of the article, he cautioned that the experiments described were "…only a 'laboratory' solution of the problem of how to make tissue homografts immunologically acceptable to hosts which would normally react against them."

Massive radiation exposures provided an opportunity to advance therapies for bone marrow failure syndromes and leukemia. A series of critical studies in mice, dogs, and subsequently nonhuman primates that were subjected to high doses of radiation followed by transplantation of marrow grafts provided the basis for understanding concepts of histocompatibility, conditioning, graft-versus-leukemia effect, and GVHD.

Jacobson and colleagues[15] reported that the shielding of spleen, part of the liver, the head, or even 1 hind leg of mice allowed survival after total body irradiation. They also demonstrated similar protection if spleen grafts were transplanted intraperitoneally immediately after radiation exposure. These investigators posited that this phenomenon could be due to "a substance of a non-cellular nature" or that irradiation produced a "toxin" which was "detoxified" by shielding the spleen or the grafting tissues.[15] By 1954, this "humoral" hypothesis was clearly trumped by the "cellular" hypothesis. Barnes and Louitit[16] suggested that living cells were responsible for hematopoietic recovery after radiation. Shortly thereafter, many independent investigators confirmed that after lethal radiation, hematopoietic recovery was dependent upon donor cells.[17–19]

Experienced with marrow transplant work in rodents, Mathé and colleagues[20] in France was faced with the need to rescue 5 subjects who had accidentally been exposed to high doses of radiation. He used bone marrow infusions from different donors. Of the 5 subjects, 4 survived. Subsequently it was recognized that this was because of autologous recovery. His group went on to describe early trials of adaptive immunotherapy with marrow grafts for the management of leukemia patients. Even though all patients died, complete remission from the leukemia was described for several patients for periods of 5 and 9 months before they died of either infection or the secondary disease (today known as GVHD).[21] At around the same time, Thomas and colleagues[22] in the United States attempted human bone marrow transplants for leukemia. Five subjects with end-stage malignancies were infused with marrow from fetuses and adults. These investigators made special efforts to demonstrate that all collections were free of infection and were infused safely in the subjects without immediate transfusion reactions. Unfortunately none of the patients survived. Parenthetically, they also opined that although bone marrow is a source of plasma cells, patients with agammaglobulinemia, which had been recently described by Bruton,[23,24] need not be treated with this modality because these patients did well on infusions of gamma globulin and antibiotics.[22] This remains true today, 50 years later, with the one caveat that some of these patients develop progressive and fatal encephalitis[25] that might be averted by bone marrow transplantation.

As had been previously reported, marrow grafting experiments in dogs were subject to the same consequences as noted in mice: after radiation, the animals could recover promptly if rescued with autologous marrow.[26] In contrast, when allogeneic grafts were used, the graft was rejected, indicative of the immune competence of the animal, or successful engraftment was achieved, followed by lethal GVHD. Most importantly, it was already becoming clear that successful allogeneic marrow transplants, unlike solid organ transplants, depended upon close histocompatibility matching between donor and recipient and, thus, would be limited by the availability of donors. GVHD (the former) and histocompatibility (the latter) represented two hurdles that needed to be surmounted before bone marrow transplantation could be generally applied as a therapeutic modality for many.

THE CHALLENGES OF GVHD

At the same time that these early transplants were being performed for treatment of leukemia, the classification of PIDs was being refined. Attempts to correct lymphopenia with conventional blood transfusions were unsuccessful and often fatal.[27] In 1967, the first symposium on the immunologic deficiencies in man took place in Sanibel Island, Florida.[28] Severe combined immunodeficiency (SCID), until then divided into Swiss type agammaglobulinemia (ie, autosomal recessive) or sex-linked lymphopenic immunologic deficiency, was attributed to thymic dysfunction. However, unlike the situation in DiGeorge syndrome, thymus transplants in SCID were not corrective. DeVries and colleagues[29] suggested that the thymus defect might be secondary and hypothesized that the absence of lymphoid progenitors was the root cause of the combined defect. It made sense then to reconstitute such SCID infants with a source of lymphoid precursors, such as spleen, fetal liver, and bone marrow. Thus, in contrast to patients with leukemia, the main barrier was not rejection of the graft or relapse of leukemia, it was the terrible secondary disease or GVHD (**Fig. 1**).

In August of 1968, an editorial was published by Hong and colleagues,[30] outlining the hazards and potential benefits of blood transfusions in immunologic deficiencies. It was proposed that either "old blood" or irradiated blood products be used in

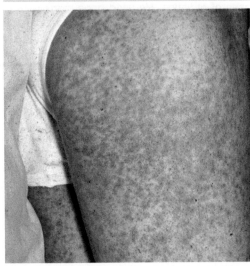

Graft-versus-Host Reaction

Fig. 1. GVHD in a patient who developed fever, maculopapular rash, hepatosplenomegaly, pancytopenia, and death.

severely immunodeficient patients as a means of preventing GVHD. These authors further hypothesized that if one could find a histocompatible match, the immunologic capacity of the immunodeficient host could potentially be restored.

The first HLA antigens in man were described by Dausset[31] in France, van Rood and colleagues[32] in Holland, Payne and Rolfs[33] and Amos[34,35] in the United States, and Ceppellini and van Rood[36] in Italy. Terasaki and McClellan[37] had developed methodology for a rapidly expanding panel of HLA antigens. A second HLA-Class I locus (HLA-B) had not yet been fully appreciated, most likely because of the high degree of linkage disequilibrium between the closely linked HLA-A and B loci (ie, 1 cM). Continuing studies in mice and dogs consistently demonstrated that if animals were well matched, GVHD could be prevented.[38–40] Occasionally mild reactions occurred, but these were thought to be transient.

With this background of imperfect but rapidly developing knowledge, including the experience being accrued by oncologists,[22,41] a window in history opened when the "right" patient was referred to Robert A. Good, then at the University of Minnesota (discussed in the next section).

RENEWED HOPE FOR SCID PATIENTS

In the late 1950s, X-linked SCID was described (today known as common gamma chain–deficient SCID or γc-SCID). Most likely, this combined immunodeficiency is severe because the defective γ-chain is common to 5 interleukin (IL) receptors (IL-2, IL-7, IL-9, IL-15, and IL-21). Children with this disorder would come to medical attention early in life and die shortly thereafter with recurring and finally overwhelming infections, such as persistent thrush, fatal pneumonias, vaccinia gangrenosa, and susceptibility to *Pneumocystis*. In Sweden at that time, bacille Calmette-Guérin

(BCG) vaccination for tuberculosis was mandatory, and about a dozen deaths were recognized related to this immunologic deficiency.[42]

A 5-month-old male child was referred to the University of Minnesota. The baby had previously been diagnosed in Boston as having "thymic alymphoplasia and agammaglobulinemia" (or X-linked SCID). The family history was significant for 11 male deaths over 3 generations. All had died of infections in early infancy (**Fig. 2**).[43] The patient had low serum gamma globulins and was being treated with gamma globulin injections and antibiotics for persistent pneumonia. A chest radiograph revealed absence of thymus. Hematologic studies noted lymphopenia. Antibodies against blood group antigens, diphtheria toxoid, and typhoid antigens were not detected. Cellular responses were absent. Tonsils, adenoids, and peripheral lymph nodes could not be detected.[44]

The most hopeful piece of information was that the child had 4 sisters, for this increased the chances of finding a matched sibling for marrow transplantation. Two forms of histocompatibility testing were developing at the time: (1) serologic typing for HLA (Class I only) and (2) cellular typing by mixed leukocyte cultures (MLCs).

HLA typing was performed by Terasaki at the University of California, Los Angeles. Of all sisters analyzed, 1 was found to be the best match. MLCs, performed by Meuwissen[45] in Minneapolis, demonstrated reactivity to the patient's cells in all 4 sisters; however, 1 sister (sister 3) clearly had a weak reaction (**Fig. 3**). This sister was also ABO incompatible. Making sense of the histocompatibility testing results at that time was a source of considerable discussion and soul-searching, for a misinterpretation of the genetics or biology could result in fatal GVHD reaction: (1) the HLA antigens did not segregate and (2) they did not seem to correlate with the segregation of the MLC results. Only after it was appreciated several years later that 2 serologic loci (HLA-A and HLA-B) existed could a crossover between the 2 loci in the donor cells be postulated to explain the serologic typing.[46] And only when the Class II loci were localized proximal to the Class I region of the MHC on chromosome 6 could one

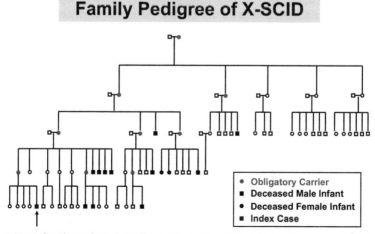

Fig. 2. Patient family pedigree. (*Adapted from* Good RA. Immunologic reconstitution: the achievement and it's meaning. In: Bergsma D, Good RA, editors. Birth defects original articles series, vol. 4. White Plains (NY): The National Foundation-March of Dimes; 1968; with permission.)

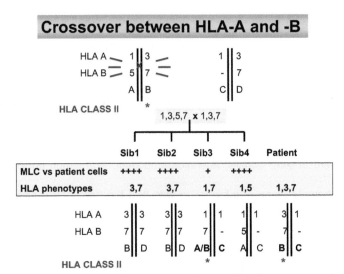

Fig. 3. Histocompatibility testing of an X-SCID patient and family members, using HLA serologic typing and unidirectional MLC. Note that segregation of both HLA haplotyping and MLC reactions were only understandable after a crossover between HLA-A and HLA-B loci was appreciated. Class II loci on haplotype B (*asterisks*) of the patient would have then segregated with the proximal portion of recombinant haplotype B in Sib3, who became the stem cell donor. (*Data from* Gatti RA, Meuwissen HJ, Terasaki PI, et al. Recombination within the HL-A locus. Tissue Antigens 1971;1(5):239–41.)

postulate that the crossover between HLA-A and HLA-B in sister 3 would carry with it the Class II region shared between patient and donor on haplotype B (see **Fig. 3**).

Driven by the almost certain fatal outcome of the disease in this family without treatment, a decision was made to attempt the bone marrow transplant using the 8-year-old sister 3 as the donor.[44] Both peripheral blood and bone marrow (obtained from iliac crests and tibial bones) were collected from the donor. Peripheral blood was collected 48 hours before collecting the marrow so that a stem-cell–rich fraction of nucleated cells could be prepared by density gradient centrifugation using 5% dextran. The cells were resuspended in donor plasma. In contrast to what was being done for oncologic patients, the infusion of both peripheral blood (5×10^6 lymphocytes/mL) and marrow (total of 10^9 nucleated cells) was given intraperitoneally, primarily to avoid having to filter out bone spicules and thereby reduce the number of cells available for engraftment. (In today's terms, approximately 10×10^6 CD34$^+$ cells were infused into the 7-kg infant, or 1.25×10^6 stem cells/kg.)

One week after the cells were infused, GVHD symptoms appeared, involving the skin, gut, and liver. This was accompanied by a hemolytic anemia thought to be caused by donor/host ABO incompatibility. No immunosuppressive therapies were given because of concern that immunosuppressive drugs would impede stem cell engraftment and because of experimental evidence that a mild GVHD would subside. One week later, the high fever and rash disappeared, and engraftment ensued. Proliferative responses to mitogens normalized, delayed-type hypersensitivity reactions could be demonstrated for the first time, and a bone marrow aspirate showed that 25% of bone marrow cells could be identified as female (donor) by karyotyping.

Despite this early success, 45 days later, the patient developed a severe aplastic anemia. It was speculated that this was GVHD reaction involving the marrow.

Donor-specific cytotoxic antibodies were demonstrated. A second bone marrow infusion followed.[45,47] Within 2 weeks, the leukocyte counts improved, GVHD had subsided, and the proportion of erythrocytes with the host's group A type had begun to decline, shifting instead to the donor's group O blood type.[47] Group O cells have persisted to date, and the patient remains cured from his SCID diagnosis. For the first time, both SCID and aplastic anemia had been corrected by bone marrow transplantation and new therapeutic options became available for these disorders. It is also important to recognize that this experience confirmed the proposed model that the central defect in SCID patients resided in their lack of pluripotent stem cells and not a defective thymic microenvironment. A 2-year posttransplant evaluation demonstrated not only a stable immunologic reconstitution but also the transfer of T-cell memory, as evidenced by positive skin tests to mumps, despite that the child had never had mumps; the donor had had mumps shortly before her cells were harvested for transplant.

Bach and colleagues[48] described a 22-month-old boy who was engrafted with bone marrow from a sister to correct for Wiskott-Aldrich syndrome (WAS). In contrast to patients with SCID, patients with WAS have evidence of immunologic function. To overcome the potential for rejection, a conditioning regimen consisting of azathioprine (5 mg/kg) and prednisone (2 mg/kg) was given for 2 days before the transplant. In contrast to the SCID case, the marrow infusion (6.5×10^9) was given intravenously through a femoral line. The patient developed *Staphylococcus aureus* positive intravenous line sepsis and graft failure. A second bone marrow transplant was given 4 days later, consisting of donor-derived peripheral blood mononuclear cells (PBMCs). It was speculated that donor PBMCs induced the expansion of recipient lymphocytes against minor donor HLA antigens. These lymphocytes would be subsequently eliminated by successive doses of cyclophosphamide at specific intervals. The transplanted female marrow initially seemed to engraft successfully. Fifteen years later, the patient was noted to have full T-cell and partial B-cell chimerism but no evidence of hematopoietic engraftment and remained thrombocytopenic.[49]

THE DARK DAYS AND THE DRAWING BOARD

Despite early enthusiasm, the reality was that transplantation for anything other than severe immunodeficiency seemed to be of limited clinical application. An excellent review of all bone marrow transplants attempted between 1939 to 1969 was carefully recorded by Mortimer Bortin.[50] The cases included 73 patients with aplastic anemia, 84 with leukemia, 31 with malignant disease, and 15 with immunodeficiency. Radiation and chloramphenicol were the most important known causes for aplastic anemia. Sixty percent of patients with acute leukemias were children (<18 years). Seven percent of autopsies had pulmonary evidence of marrow emboli. Of 203 transplants, at the time the report was written, 152 patients had died. Taken together, in 125 patients (60%) there was no evidence of engraftment. Evidence of chimerism was recognized in 11. Only 3 patients survived (all were immunodeficient patients and included the 2 patients described earlier). Graft rejection, infection, and GVHD were the main causes of death.

During the 1970s, donor selection, control of GVHD, and conditioning regimens became areas of intense research in preclinical models. MLCs were used for the selection of donors. Weak in vitro responses suggested good compatibility. However, as HLA typing improved, it became apparent that MLC assays were difficult to interpret and were less reliable than what was required for clinical application. Serological testing for HLA-class II antigens was instituted. By the turn of the century serology was largely replaced by molecular identification of histocompatibility antigens. By 1975, Thomas and colleagues[51] published the first of a 2-part medical progress report on bone marrow transplantation. In this excellent synopsis, the authors discussed animal studies, the status of histocompatibility testing, conditioning regimens, techniques for marrow collection, fractionation and infusion, and the level of supportive care necessary for successful bone marrow transplantation.[52,53]

DECADES OF ADVANCES

The 1980s and 1990s saw a rapid increase in the number of transplants performed; national and international bone marrow registries were created, and cord blood was recognized as a source of stem cells. T-cell depletion techniques were introduced for prevention of GVHD, as matched sibling donors were only available 25% of the time, whereas HLA-haploidentical or mismatched family members were readily available. Soybean lectin agglutination coupled with erythrocyte rosetting with sheep red blood cell was developed by Reisner and colleagues[54] and was used successfully in patients with SCID and subsequently in patients with leukemia. Since that time, this approach has allowed for the survival of many infants with SCID[55–58] and continues to be used today in different centers around the world.

Novel methods of T-cell depletion were developed, including counterflow centrifugal elutriation and fractionation on density gradients.[59,60] By 1981, the first clinical trial using antithymocyte globulin was reported.[61] Subsequently monoclonal antibodies were used in vivo and ex vivo for the treatment of marrow grafts for malignancies and PID patients.[62–65] However, with the depletion of T cells, important complications were recognized. These complications were higher incidence of graft failures, delayed immune reconstitution, increased risk of Epstein-Bar virus–associated lymphoproliferative disease, and CMV reactivation, and the overall survival was not significantly improved as compared with non–T-cell-depleted bone marrow.[66]

When CD34 was recognized as a glycoprotein that helped to identify hematopoietic progenitor cells, their isolation from peripheral blood provided another stem cell source. These peripheral blood stem cells (PBSCs) are capable of forming colonies of granulocytes/macrophages, erythrocytes, and other multipotential or immature progenitors.[67] The introduction of growth factors such as granulocyte colony-stimulating factor(filgrastim) and granulocyte/macrophage colony-stimulating factor (sargramostim), plerixafor[68] (a novel molecule that inhibits chemokine receptor CXCR4 binding to stromal cell–derived factor-1), and other agents[69] have contributed to successful mobilization of CD34$^+$ cells into the peripheral circulation and thus their use as a source of hematopoietic stem cells (HSCs). These PBSCs permitted high-dose salvage therapy to patients with refractory malignancies, resulting in prolonged survival and impeding tumor progression.[70] Although PBSCs have become a common source of HSCs for autologous transplants, their role in allogeneic transplants is still unclear.[71–73] Use of PBSCs may be influenced by multiple factors, including preference of the transplant center, primary disease, risk of relapse, graft-versus-leukemia effect, and donor preference. Experience with PBSCs for transplantation in patients with PID is limited.

Umbilical cord blood (UCB) represents another alternative source of HSCs and has become a standard option for both children and adults with hematopoietic disorders and malignancies.[74,75] The advantages include (1) a low rate of viral contamination, (2) lower rates of GVHD, and (3) readily available units.[76] The use of UCB for PID is limited. However 2 single-center experiences have been reported.[77,78] In both series, immunologic reconstitution was demonstrated.

Another promising methodology for HSCT would be to downregulate HLA expression by genetically engineering donor cells, using RNA interference (RNA$_i$). This enables the cells to evade immune recognition.[79] By integrating RNA$_i$ into genomic DNA, a universally accepted and expandable pool of donor cells would become available.

CURRENT STATUS OF SCT FOR PID

There is no doubt that, for the past 4 decades, allogeneic SCT for PID has allowed for survival of patients in whom the natural history of the disease predicted an early death. The Center for International Blood and Marrow Transplant Research (CIBMTR) collects data in collaboration with the European Groups for Blood and Marrow Transplantation (EBMT), the Asia-Pacific Blood Marrow Transplant group (APBMT), and the World Marrow Donor Association (WMDA) along with transplants performed in North and South America. A progress report of comprehensive data as of 2008 is available, including more than 1500 transplants performed around the world for patients with SCID and other PIDs.[2]

SCID represents the group of patients for whom HSCT is now considered standard of care; indeed, this PID has achieved the most successful survival record ranging from 63% to 100% when an HLA-matched sibling donor is available and 50% to 77% when haploidentical or HLA-mismatched donors are used.[58,80–87] The lack of donor availability, variable evidence of long-term immunologic reconstitution, and other limitations have led to the extensive use of unrelated but matched donors as a source of stem cells for SCID. The outcomes have improved over the recent years, with survivals ranging from 63% to 80%.[81,84,85,87,88]

The largest groups of non-SCID patients with primary immunodeficiencies for which SCT has been successful include WAS and chronic granulomatous disease. A collaborative study of the International Bone Marrow Transplant registry analyzed 170 transplants performed for WAS between 1968 and 1996. The overall 5-year probability of survival was 70% (95% confidence interval [CI], 63%–77%). Best outcomes were noted for patients receiving transplants from an HLA-identical sibling, 87% (95% CI, 74%–93%) as compared with 52% (95% CI, 37%–65%) for those receiving from other related donors. Matched unrelated donor transplants demonstrated a 5-year probability of survival of 71% (95% CI, 58%–80%). Of interest, if children receiving matched unrelated donor transplants were transplanted before the age of 5 years, the outcome was similar to HLA-matched sibling transplants.[89]

A more recent long-term outcome analysis for patients who underwent transplant for WAS was performed by the European Society for Immunodeficiencies (ESID) and the EBMT.[90] Included in the study were patients who had survived at least 2 years after HSCT. Survival was similar: 7-year event-free survival of 75%. Yet, a 20% incidence of autoimmunity was associated with mixed chimerism, independent of chronic GVHD. Furthermore, infection related to splenectomy was identified as an iatrogenic complication.[90]

Chronic granulomatous disease, an inherited disease of neutrophil function, is conventionally treated with prophylactic antibiotics and/or interferon therapy.[91] However, long-term follow-up data suggest significant morbidity caused by infection and only 50% to 55% survival through the third and forth decades of life.[92,93] HSCT has been a therapeutic option for the past 2 decades.[94,95] In 2002, the EBMT group reported results of 27 transplants from 1985 to 2000. Almost all (22 of 23) patients survived. These patients had received a myeloablative busulfan-containing conditioning regimen from an HLA-identical donor and achieved full and stable donor chimerism.[96] More recently, excellent survival (90%) after HSCT has been reported by the Newcastle group, with a median 61 months of follow-up.[97]

Disorders such as X-linked lymphoproliferative syndrome,[98] the familial forms of hemophagocytic lymphohistiocytosis,[99] leukocyte adhesion deficiency,[100] CD40 ligand deficiency,[101,102] and immunodysregulation polyendocrinopathy enteropathy X-linked syndrome[103] are within the spectrum of diseases treated with HSCT. Patients with Chédiak-Higashi syndrome have also been treated with HSCT; however, late-onset cognitive impairment has been described 20 years posttransplant.[104]

SUMMARY

The last 40 years has seen the emergence of HSCT as a therapeutic modality for fatal diseases and as a curative option for individuals born with inherited disorders that carry limited life expectancy and poor quality of life. Despite the rarity of many PIDs, these disorders have led the way toward innovative therapies and further provide insights into mechanisms of immunologic reconstitution applicable to all HSC transplants. Critical analysis of outcomes and prospective multicenter clinical trials will be necessary to further our understanding as to best therapeutic approaches for patients with PID, who constitute a very heterogenous group of patients.

REFERENCES

1. Bekkum DW, van de Vries MJ. Radiation chimaeras. London: Logos Press; 1967. p. 277.
2. The Medical College of Wisconsin and The National Marrow Donor Program. Center for International Blood and Marrow Transplant Research (CIBMTR). Available at: http://www.cibmtr.org/. 2008. Accessed October 28, 2009.
3. Good RA, Kapoor N, Reisner Y. Bone marrow transplantation—an expanding approach to treatment of many diseases. Cell Immunol 1983;82(1):36–54.
4. Quine WME. The remedial application of bone marrow. JAMA 1896;26:1012.
5. Tiselius A, Kabat EA. An electrophoretic study of immune sera and purified antibody preparations. J Exp Med 1939;69:119–31.
6. White TF, Dougherty A. Functional alterations in lymphoid tissue induced by adrenal cortical secretion. Am J Anat 1945;77:81–116.
7. Medawar PB. The experimental study of skin grafts. Br Med Bull 1945;3:79.
8. Owen R. Immunogenetic consequences of vascular anastomoses between bovine twins. Science 1945;28:400.
9. Loeb L. Heredity and internal secretion in the spontaneous development of cancer in mice. Science 1915;42(1095):912–4.
10. Gorer PA. The detection of antigenic differences in mouse erythrocytes by employment of immune sera. Br J Exp Pathol 1936;17:21.
11. Snell GD, Stevens LC. Histocompatibility genes of mice. III. H-1 and H-4, two histocompatibility loci in the first linkage group. Immunology 1961;4:366–79.
12. Snell GD. Histocompatibility genes of the mouse. I. Demonstration of weak histocompatibility differences by immunization and controlled tumor dosage. J Natl Cancer Inst 1958;20(4):787–824.
13. Snell GD, Jackson RB. Histocompatibility genes of the mouse. II. Production and analysis of isogenic resistant lines. J Natl Cancer Inst 1958;21(5):843–77.
14. Billingham RE, Brent L, Medawar PB. Actively acquired tolerance of foreign cells. Nature 1953;172:603–6.
15. Jacobson LO, Simmons EL, Marks EK, et al. Recovery from radiation injury. Science 1951;113:510–1.

16. Barnes DW, Ford CE, Ilbery PL, et al. Tissue transplantation in the radiation chimera. J Cell Physiol Suppl 1957;50(Suppl 1):123–38.
17. Main JM, Prehn RT. Successful skin homografts after the administration of high dosage X radiation and homologous bone marrow. J Natl Cancer Inst 1955; 15(4):1023–9.
18. Ford CE, Hamerton JL, Barnes DW, et al. Cytological identification of radiation-chimaeras. Nature 1956;177(4506):452–4.
19. Crouch BG, Overman RR. Chemical protection against x-radiation death in primates: a preliminary report. Science 1957;125(3257):1092.
20. Mathé G, Jammet H, Pendie N, et al. Transfusions et greffes de moelle osseuse homologue chez des humaine irradies a haute dose accidentellement. Nouvelle rev franc hematol 1959;4:226.
21. Mathe G, Amiel JL, Schwarzenberg L, et al. Adoptive immunotherapy of acute leukemia: experimental and clinical results. Cancer Res 1965;25(9):1525–31.
22. Thomas ED, Lochte HL Jr, Lu WC, et al. Intravenous infusion of bone marrow in patients receiving radiation and chemotherapy. N Engl J Med 1957;257(11): 491–6.
23. Bruton OC. Agammaglobulinemia. Pediatrics 1952;9(6):722–8.
24. Bruton OC, Apt L, Gitlin D, et al. Absence of serum gamma globulins. AMA Am J Dis Child 1952;84(5):632–6.
25. Medici MA, Kagan RM, Menkes J, et al. Chronic progressive panencephalitis in hypogammaglobulinemia: a literature review. In: JMR Foundation, editor. Immunodeficiency. Its nature and etiological significance in human diseases. Tokyo: University of Tokyo Press; 1978. p. 149–60.
26. Mannick JA, Lochte HL Jr, Ashley CA, et al. Autografts of bone marrow in dogs after lethal total-body radiation. Blood 1960;15:255–66.
27. Miller ME. Thymic dysplasia ("Swiss agammaglobulinemia"). I. Graft versus host reaction following bone-marrow transfusion. J Pediatr 1967;70(5):730–6.
28. Bregsma D, Good RA, editors. Immunologic deficiency in man. Birth defects original articles series, vol. 4. White Plains (NY): The National Foundation-March of Dimes; 1968.
29. de Vries MJ, Dooren LJ, Cleton FJ. Graft versus host or autoimmune lesions in the Swiss type of agammaglobulinemia. In: Bergsma D, editor. Immunologic Deficiency in Man. Birth defects original articles series, vol. 4. White Plains (NY): National Foundation-March of Dimes; 1968. p.173.
30. Hong R, Cooper MD, Allan MJ, et al. Immunological restitution in lymphopenic immunological deficiency syndrome. Lancet 1968;1(7541):503–6.
31. Dausset J. [Presence of A & B antigens in leukocytes disclosed by agglutination tests]. C R Seances Soc Biol Fil 1954;148(19–20):1607–8 [in French].
32. van Rood JJ, van Leeuwen A, van Santen MC. Anti HL-A2 inhibitor in normal human serum. Nature 1970;226(5243):366–7.
33. Payne R, Rolfs MR. Fetomaternal leukocyte incompatibility. J Clin Invest 1958; 37(12):1756–63.
34. Amos DB. Genetic and antigenetic aspects of human histocompatibility systems. Adv Immunol 1969;10:251–97.
35. Amos DB, Seigler HF, Southworth JG, et al. Skin graft rejection between subjects genotyped for HL-A. Transplant Proc 1969;1(1):342–6.
36. Ceppellini R, van Rood JJ. The HL-A system. I. Genetics and molecular biology. Semin Hematol 1974;11(3):233–51.
37. Terasaki PI, McClelland JD. Microdroplet assay of human serum cytotoxins. Nature 1964;204:998–1000.

38. Simonsen M. Graft versus host reactions. Their natural history, and applicability as tools of research. Prog Allergy 1962;6:349–467.

39. Good RA, Martinez C, Gabrielsen AE. Progress toward transplantation of tissues in man. Adv Pediatr 1964;13:93–127.

40. Storb R, Epstein RB, Bryant J, et al. Marrow grafts by combined marrow and leukocyte infusions in unrelated dogs selected by histocompatibility typing. Transplantation 1968;6(4):587–93.

41. Thomas ED, Epstein RB, Eschbach JW Jr, et al. Treatment of leukemia by extra-corporeal irradiation. N Engl J Med 1965;273:6–12.

42. Good RA, Fisher DW. In: Good RA, Fisher DW, editors. Immunobiology: current knowledge of basic concepts in immunology and their clinical applications. Stamford (CT): Sinauer Associates; 1971. p. 305.

43. Good RA. Immunologic reconstitution: the achievement and it's meaning. In: Bergsma D, Good RA, editors. Birth defects original articles series, vol. 4. White Plains (NY): The National Foundation-March of Dimes; 1968.

44. Gatti RA, Meuwissen HJ, Allen HD, et al. Immunological reconstitution of sex-linked lymphopenic immunological deficiency. Lancet 1968;2(7583):1366–9.

45. Meuwissen HJ, Gatti RA, Terasaki PI, et al. Treatment of lymphopenic hypogamma-globulinemia and bone-marrow aplasia by transplantation of allogeneic marrow. Crucial role of histocompatibility matching. N Engl J Med 1969;281(13):691–7.

46. Gatti RA, Meuwissen HJ, Terasaki PI, et al. Recombination within the HL-A locus. Tissue Antigens 1971;1(5):239–41.

47. Gatti RA, Good RA. Follow-up of correction of severe dual system immunodefi-ciency with bone marrow transplantation. J Pediatr 1971;79(3):475–9.

48. Bach FH, Albertini RJ, Joo P, et al. Bone-marrow transplantation in a patient with the Wiskott-Aldrich syndrome. Lancet 1968;2(7583):1364–6.

49. Meuwissen HJ, Bortin MM, Bach FH, et al. Long-term survival after bone marrow transplantation: a 15-year follow-up report of a patient with Wiskott-Aldrich syndrome. J Pediatr 1984;105(3):365–9.

50. Bortin MM. A compendium of reported human bone marrow transplants. Trans-plantation 1970;9(6):571–87.

51. Thomas ED, Storb R, Clift RA, et al. Bone-marrow transplantation (second of two parts). N Engl J Med 1975;292(17):895–902.

52. Gatti RA, Kemple K, Schwartzmann J, et al. HLA-D typing with lymphoblastoid cell lines. VI. Rationale and goals of data reduction. Tissue Antigens 1979;14(3): 183–93.

53. Gatti RA, Kempner DH, Leibold W. The role of the MHC antigens in the mature and immature host. Pediatrics 1979;64(5 Pt 2 Suppl):803–13.

54. Reisner Y, Kapoor N, Kirkpatrick D, et al. Transplantation for severe combined immunodeficiency with HLA-A, B, D, DR incompatible parental marrow cells fractionated by soybean agglutinin and sheep red blood cells. Blood 1983; 61(2):341–8.

55. O'Reilly RJ, Keever CA, Small TN, et al. The use of HLA-non-identical T-cell-depleted marrow transplants for correction of severe combined immunodefi-ciency disease. Immunodefic Rev 1989;1(4):273–309.

56. Buckley RH, Schiff SE, Sampson HA, et al. Development of immunity in human severe primary T cell deficiency following haploidentical bone marrow stem cell transplantation. J Immunol 1986;136(7):2398–407.

57. Dror Y, Gallagher R, Wara DW, et al. Immune reconstitution in severe combined immunodeficiency disease after lectin-treated, T-cell-depleted haplocompatible bone marrow transplantation. Blood 1993;81(8):2021–30.

58. Buckley RH, Schiff SE, Schiff RI, et al. Hematopoietic stem-cell transplantation for the treatment of severe combined immunodeficiency. N Engl J Med 1999; 340(7):508–16.
59. de Witte T, Hoogenhout J, de Pauw B, et al. Depletion of donor lymphocytes by counterflow centrifugation successfully prevents acute graft-versus-host disease in matched allogeneic marrow transplantation. Blood 1986;67(5):1302–8.
60. Lowenberg B, Wagemaker G, van Bekkum DW, et al. Graft-versus-host disease following transplantation of 'one log' versus 'two log' T-lymphocyte-depleted bone marrow from HLA-identical donors. Bone Marrow Transplant 1986;1(2): 133–40.
61. Rodt H, Kolb HJ, Netzel B, et al. Effect of anti-T-cell globulin on GVHD in leukemic patients treated with BMT. Transplant Proc 1981;13(1 Pt 1):257–61.
62. Filipovich AH, McGlave P, Ramsay NK, et al. Treatment of donor bone marrow with OKT3 (PAN-T monoclonal antibody) for prophylaxis of graft-vs.-host disease (GvHD) in histocompatible allogeneic bone marrow transplantation (BMT): a pilot study. J Clin Immunol 1982;2(Suppl 3):154S–7S.
63. Filipovich AH, McGlave PB, Ramsay NK, et al. Pretreatment of donor bone marrow with monoclonal antibody OKT3 for prevention of acute graft-versus-host disease in allogeneic histocompatible bone-marrow transplantation. Lancet 1982;1(8284):1266–9.
64. Martin PJ, Hansen JA, Thomas ED. Preincubation of donor bone marrow cells with a combination of murine monoclonal anti-T-cell antibodies without complement does not prevent graft-versus-host disease after allogeneic marrow transplantation. J Clin Immunol 1984;4(1):18–22.
65. Umiel T, Daley JF, Bhan AK, et al. Acquisition of immune competence by a subset of human cortical thymocytes expressing mature T cell antigens. J Immunol 1982;129(3):1054–60.
66. Ho VT, Soiffer RJ. The history and future of T-cell depletion as graft-versus-host disease prophylaxis for allogeneic hematopoietic stem cell transplantation. Blood 2001;98(12):3192–204.
67. Krause DS, Fackler MJ, Civin CI, et al. CD34: structure, biology, and clinical utility. Blood 1996;87(1):1–13.
68. Cashen AF. Plerixafor hydrochloride: a novel agent for the mobilization of peripheral blood stem cells. Drugs Today (Barc) 2009;45(7):497–505.
69. Greinix HT, Worel N. New agents for mobilizing peripheral blood stem cells. Transfus Apher Sci 2009;41(1):67–71.
70. Kessinger A, Armitage JO, Smith DM, et al. High-dose therapy and autologous peripheral blood stem cell transplantation for patients with lymphoma. Blood 1989;74(4):1260–5.
71. Pidala J, Anasetti C, Kharfan-Dabaja MA, et al. Decision analysis of peripheral blood versus bone marrow hematopoietic stem cells for allogeneic hematopoietic cell transplantation. Biol Blood Marrow Transplant 2009;15(11): 1415–21.
72. Gallardo D, de la Camara R, Nieto JB, et al. Is mobilized peripheral blood comparable with bone marrow as a source of hematopoietic stem cells for allogeneic transplantation from HLA-identical sibling donors? A case-control study. Haematologica 2009;94(9):1282–8.
73. Gorin NC, Labopin M, Blaise D, et al. Higher incidence of relapse with peripheral blood rather than marrow as a source of stem cells in adults with acute myelocytic leukemia autografted during the first remission. J Clin Oncol 2009; 27(24):3987–93.

74. Gluckman E, Broxmeyer HA, Auerbach AD, et al. Hematopoietic reconstitution in a patient with Fanconi's anemia by means of umbilical-cord blood from an HLA-identical sibling. N Engl J Med 1989;321(17):1174–8.

75. Gluckman E, Rocha V, Boyer-Chammard A, et al. Outcome of cord-blood transplantation from related and unrelated donors. Eurocord Transplant Group and the European Blood and Marrow Transplantation Group. N Engl J Med 1997; 337(6):373–81.

76. Gluckman E, Rocha V. Cord blood transplantation: state of the art. Haematologica 2009;94(4):451–4.

77. Knutsen AP, Wall DA. Umbilical cord blood transplantation in severe T-cell immunodeficiency disorders: two-year experience. J Clin Immunol 2000;20(6):466–76.

78. Bhattacharya A, Slatter MA, Chapman CE, et al. Single centre experience of umbilical cord stem cell transplantation for primary immunodeficiency. Bone Marrow Transplant 2005;36(4):295–9.

79. Hacke K, Falahati R, Flebbe-Rehwaldt L, et al. Suppression of HLA expression by lentivirus-mediated gene transfer of siRNA cassettes and in vivo chemoselection to enhance hematopoietic stem cell transplantation. Immunol Res 2009;44(1–3):112–26.

80. Fischer A, Landais P, Friedrich W, et al. Bone marrow transplantation (BMT) in Europe for primary immunodeficiencies other than severe combined immunodeficiency: a report from the European Group for BMT and the European Group for Immunodeficiency. Blood 1994;83(4):1149–54.

81. Antoine C, Muller S, Cant A, et al. Long-term survival and transplantation of haemopoietic stem cells for immunodeficiencies: report of the European experience 1968-99. Lancet 2003;361(9357):553–60.

82. Patel NC, Chinen J, Rosenblatt HM, et al. Long-term outcomes of nonconditioned patients with severe combined immunodeficiency transplanted with HLA-identical or haploidentical bone marrow depleted of T cells with anti-CD6 mAb. J Allergy Clin Immunol 2008;122(6):1185–93.

83. Haddad E, Landais P, Friedrich W, et al. Long-term immune reconstitution and outcome after HLA-nonidentical T-cell-depleted bone marrow transplantation for severe combined immunodeficiency: a European retrospective study of 116 patients. Blood 1998;91(10):3646–53.

84. Roifman CM, Grunebaum E, Dalal I, et al. Matched unrelated bone marrow transplant for severe combined immunodeficiency. Immunol Res 2007; 38(1–3):191–200.

85. Grunebaum E, Mazzolari E, Porta F, et al. Bone marrow transplantation for severe combined immune deficiency. JAMA 2006;295(5):508–18.

86. Railey MD, Lokhnygina Y, Buckley RH. Long-term clinical outcome of patients with severe combined immunodeficiency who received related donor bone marrow transplants without pretransplant chemotherapy or post-transplant GVHD prophylaxis. J Pediatr 2009;155(6):834–40, e1.

87. Mazzolari E, Forino C, Guerci S, et al. Long-term immune reconstitution and clinical outcome after stem cell transplantation for severe T-cell immunodeficiency. J Allergy Clin Immunol 2007;120(4):892–9.

88. Rao K, Amrolia PJ, Jones A, et al. Improved survival after unrelated donor bone marrow transplantation in children with primary immunodeficiency using a reduced-intensity conditioning regimen. Blood 2005;105(2):879–85.

89. Filipovich AH, Stone JV, Tomany SC, et al. Impact of donor type on outcome of bone marrow transplantation for Wiskott-Aldrich syndrome: collaborative study

of the International Bone Marrow Transplant Registry and the National Marrow Donor Program. Blood 2001;97(6):1598–603.

90. Ozsahin H, Cavazzana-Calvo M, Notarangelo LD, et al. Long-term outcome following hematopoietic stem-cell transplantation in Wiskott-Aldrich syndrome: collaborative study of the European Society for Immunodeficiencies and European Group for Blood and Marrow Transplantation. Blood 2008;111(1): 439–45.

91. The International Chronic Cooperative Study Group. A controlled trial of interferon gamma to prevent infection in chronic granulomatous disease. The International Chronic Granulomatous Disease Cooperative Study Group. N Engl J Med 1991;324(8):509–16.

92. Liese J, Kloos S, Jendrossek V, et al. Long-term follow-up and outcome of 39 patients with chronic granulomatous disease. J Pediatr 2000;137(5):687–93.

93. Jones LB, McGrogan P, Flood TJ, et al. Special article: chronic granulomatous disease in the United Kingdom and Ireland: a comprehensive national patient-based registry. Clin Exp Immunol 2008;152(2):211–8.

94. Di Bartolomeo P, Di Girolamo G, Angrilli F, et al. Reconstitution of normal neutrophil function in chronic granulomatous disease by bone marrow transplantation. Bone Marrow Transplant 1989;4(6):695–700.

95. Schettini F, De Mattia D, Manzionna MM, et al. Bone marrow transplantation for chronic granulomatous disease associated with cytochrome B deficiency. Pediatr Hematol Oncol 1987;4(3):277–9.

96. Seger RA, Gungor T, Belohradsky BH, et al. Treatment of chronic granulomatous disease with myeloablative conditioning and an unmodified hemopoietic allograft: a survey of the European experience, 1985-2000. Blood 2002;100(13): 4344–50.

97. Soncini E, Slatter MA, Jones LB, et al. Unrelated donor and HLA-identical sibling haematopoietic stem cell transplantation cure chronic granulomatous disease with good long-term outcome and growth. Br J Haematol 2009; 145(1):73–83.

98. Hoffmann T, Heilmann C, Madsen HO, et al. Matched unrelated allogeneic bone marrow transplantation for recurrent malignant lymphoma in a patient with X-linked lymphoproliferative disease (XLP). Bone Marrow Transplant 1998;22(6):603–4.

99. Jordan MB, Filipovich AH. Hematopoietic cell transplantation for hemophagocytic lymphohistiocytosis: a journey of a thousand miles begins with a single (big) step. Bone Marrow Transplant 2008;42(7):433–7.

100. Qasim W, Cavazzana-Calvo M, Davies EG, et al. Allogeneic hematopoietic stem-cell transplantation for leukocyte adhesion deficiency. Pediatrics 2009; 123(3):836–40.

101. Isam H, Al-Wahadneh A. Successful bone marrow transplantation in a child with X-linked hyper-IgM syndrome. Saudi J Kidney Dis Transpl 2004;15(4):489–93.

102. Duplantier JE, Seyama K, Day NK, et al. Immunologic reconstitution following bone marrow transplantation for X-linked hyper IgM syndrome. Clin Immunol 2001;98(3):313–8.

103. Rao A, Kamani N, Filipovich A, et al. Successful bone marrow transplantation for IPEX syndrome after reduced-intensity conditioning. Blood 2007;109(1):383–5.

104. Tardieu M, Lacroix C, Neven B, et al. Progressive neurologic dysfunctions 20 years after allogeneic bone marrow transplantation for Chediak-Higashi syndrome. Blood 2005;106(1):40–2.

Hematopoietic Stem Cell Transplantation for Severe Combined Immune Deficiency or What the Children have Taught Us

Joel M. Rappeport, MD[a], Richard J. O'Reilly, MD[b,c,d], Neena Kapoor, MD[e,f], Robertson Parkman, MD[g,h,*]

KEYWORDS

- Severe combined immune deficiency
- Hematopoietic stem cell transplantation
- Unrelated • In utero • Gene transfer

More than 40 years ago, the first successful allogeneic hematopoietic stem cell transplantation (HSCT) was reported by Robert A. Good, MD and his colleagues[1] for a child with severe combined immunodeficiency (SCID). In the succeeding years, HSCT for SCID patients have represented only a small portion of the total number of allogeneic HSCT performed. Nevertheless, the clinical and biologic importance of the patients

This work was supported by Grant Nos. CA100265 and HL54850 from the National Institutes of Health.

[a] Department of Internal Medicine, Yale University School of Medicine, 333 Cedar Street, New Haven, CT 06510, USA

[b] Department of Pediatrics, Memorial Sloan Kettering Cancer Center, 1275 York Avenue, Box 139, New York, NY 10021, USA

[c] Pediatric Bone Marrow Transplant Service, Memorial Sloan-Kettering Cancer Center, 1275 York Avenue, New York, NY 10065, USA

[d] Pediatric Oncology Research, Memorial Sloan Kettering Cancer Center, New York, NY, USA

[e] Department of Pediatrics, University of Southern California Keck School of Medicine, Los Angeles, CA, USA

[f] Bone Marrow Transplantation Program, Division of Research Immunology/Bone Marrow Transplantation, Childrens Hospital Los Angeles, Los Angeles, 4650 Sunset Boulevard, Mail Stop 62, Los Angeles, CA 90027, USA

[g] Division of Research Immunology/BMT, and The Saban Research Institute, Childrens Hospital Los Angeles, 4650 Sunset Boulevard, Mail Stop 62, Los Angeles, CA 90027, USA

[h] Department of Pediatrics, Molecular Microbiology and Immunology, University of Southern California Keck School of Medicine, Los Angeles, CA, USA

* Corresponding author. Division of Research Immunology/BMT, and The Saban Research Institute, Childrens Hospital Los Angeles, 4650 Sunset Boulevard, Mail Stop 62, Los Angeles, CA 90027.
E-mail address: rparkman@chla.usc.edu (R. Parkman).

Immunol Allergy Clin N Am 30 (2010) 17–30
doi:10.1016/j.iac.2009.10.002
0889-8561/10/$ – see front matter
immunology.theclinics.com

transplanted for SCID has continued. SCID patients were the first to be successfully transplanted with nonsibling related bone marrow, unrelated bone marrow, T-cell depleted HSCT, and genetically corrected (gene transfer) autologous HSC.[2–5] In addition, many of the biologic insights that are now widely applied to allogeneic HSCT were first identified in the transplantation of SCID patients. Therefore, this article reviews the clinical and biologic lessons that have been learned from HSCT for SCID patients, and how the information has impacted the general field of allogeneic HSCT.

PRELUDES

In 1956 it was established that rodents receiving total body irradiation (TBI) could be rescued from the lethality of bone marrow failure by the infusion of histocompatible bone marrow.[6] In those studies the importance of histocompatibility for the successful rescue of the animals from lethal TBI by the prevention of graft-versus-host disease (GVHD) was identified. In the decade between the biologic reality that the transplantation of bone marrow could rescue irradiated animals and the first successful human allogeneic HSCT, clinical investigators attempted to apply the biologic principles to the treatment of patients. A sentinel event was the irradiation accident that occurred in Yugoslavia in 1959 where 6 patients, who were heavily irradiated, were subsequently treated by the infusion of either fetal liver and spleen cells or unrelated bone marrow cells.[7] No sustained donor hematopoietic engraftment was seen in any patients, although slight increases in donor-type erythrocytes were transiently seen in some patients. The patient with the highest dose of irradiation died whereas the other patients had autologous hematopoietic recovery. Other early attempts included the use of high-dose irradiation/chemotherapy and pooled allogeneic bone marrow for the treatment of related and unrelated patients with acute leukemia. Patients with aplastic anemia were infused with bone marrow from identical twins with some patients having hematopoietic improvement, but it was unclear whether their improvement in hematopoiesis was due to the HSCT or the spontaneous recovery of their underlying aplastic anemia. Many allogeneic recipients developed acute GVHD that had similarities to GVHD seen in rodents following histoincompatible transplants. Thus, clinicians were aware that histocompatibility might improve the likelihood of successful HSCT. During the 1960s, the development of serologic reagents to detect human leukocyte antigen (HLA)-A and HLA-B permitted physicians to determine the class I histocompatibility of potential donors and recipients. The development of the mixed lymphocyte culture (MLC) permitted the determination of class II histocompatibility because no antiserum to HLA-DR existed.

CLINICAL ADVANCES
Allogeneic-Related HSCT

The first successful allogeneic HSCT was a member of a kindred in which 11 male infants had died due to severe recurrent infections during the first year of life.[1] At admission, the child had draining skin pustules, no detectable lymph nodes, and lymphopenia. At that time, no phenotypic assays existed for the enumeration of T lymphocytes, but the diagnosis was confirmed by the absence of cutaneous delayed hypersensitivity as well as functional assays showing that the patient's lymphocytes did not respond to stimulation with either phytohemagglutinin (PHA) or allogeneic cells. HLA-A and -B typing indicated that the patient and a sister were HLA-B identical but differed at one HLA-A antigen; however, the sister did not respond in MLC to stimulation with the patient's cells. The patient was transplanted with a mixture of peripheral blood leukocytes and bone marrow. The cells were given intraperitoneally. A total dose of 3.5×10^8 peripheral blood leukocytes and 1×10^9 nucleated bone marrow cells were given. A week after transplantation, the patient developed an erthymatous rash, which on skin biopsy had histopathological features characteristic of GVHD. Stimulation of the patient's peripheral blood lymphocytes showed the development of large lymphoblasts with a female karyotype, indicating that the circulatory lymphocytes were now responsive to stimulation by PHA and were of donor origin. The patient was challenged with dinitrofluorobenzene and responded to skin testing, demonstrating the development of normal delayed hypersensitivity.

The patient was blood group A and the donor blood group O. The patient's anti-B titers rose, but he developed a Coomb positive hemolytic anemia. Eight weeks after HSCT the patient's platelet and granulocyte counts began to drop, and a bone marrow aspirate showed hypocellularity with both male and female cells. The patient's bone marrow progressed to complete aplasia with all cells being of donor origin.

Three months after the first transplant the patient was transplanted for the second time with 1×10^9 bone marrow cells: 20% into the right ileac marrow space and 80% intraperitoneally. The bone marrow was treated in vitro with a horse antihuman lymphoblast globulin for 2 hours before infusion. By 2 weeks there was an increase in the platelet count, and the white blood cell count began to increase. All bone marrow cells had a female karyotype.[8] The patient is now more than 40 years old, with normal immune and hematopoietic function of donor origin.

The lessons

The authors of the initial report were not able to appreciate the significance of all their clinical and laboratory observations. The patient received peripheral blood T lymphocytes as well as bone marrow cells, and it is likely that the early onset of acute GVHD was due to the large number of donor T lymphocytes given, especially considering that the donor and patient were an HLA-A mismatch. In the second transplant to reduce the probability of GVHD, they tried to reduce the number of T lymphocytes infused by (1) taking smaller bone marrow aspiration to reduce peripheral blood contamination and (2) treating the bone marrow with antiserum to remove T lymphocytes.[9] The patient did not develop any acute GVHD after the second transplant.

Subsequent animal experiments demonstrated that the efficiency of the intraperitoneal injection of HSC was approximately one-tenth that of intravenous injection. The present clinical use of the intravenous route for HSC infusion is based on the canine experiments performed by Thomas and his colleagues. The success of the initial transplants in the SCID patient was, therefore, due to the relatively large number of cells given, the small size of the patient, and the use of a HLA-B identical and MLC nonreactive donor.

The patient developed immune-mediated bone marrow aplasia, which was also seen in some other SCID patients during the 1970s. It is of interest that, although hemolytic anemia has been seen following ABO-incompatible or histoincompatible HSCT in SCID patients in more recent years, rarely has bone marrow aplasia occurred. The reason for this clinical change is unclear. The development of bone marrow aplasia, however, clearly demonstrated that immune cell-mediated events including GVHD can produce severe aplastic anemia, indicating that immunosuppression might have a role in the treatment of aplastic anemia, which was subsequently demonstrated in both animal studies and clinical trials using antithymocyte globulin and other immunosuppressive agents.[10]

The patient, in addition to being the first patient to have an immune deficiency corrected by HSCT, also represented the first successful treatment of bone marrow failure by allogeneic HSCT. No evidence of donor hematopoietic engraftment occurred following the initial transplant. It is now clear that in SCID patients, no clinically significant donor HSC engraftment occurs without some myelosuppressive therapy. However, once the immune-mediated destruction of the recipient hematopoiesis had occurred and adequate "space" had been developed, it was possible even with the intraperitoneal infusion of donor bone marrow to establish donor-derived hematopoiesis without any chemotherapy. The patient demonstrated what it took another decade to formally prove, that is, that engraftment of donor HSC requires the elimination or reduction of the number of recipient HSC to permit the engraftment of donor hematopoietic cells.[11] The present use of reduced intensity regimens that rely on the engraftment of the donor immune system to eliminate both normal and abnormal (neoplastic) recipient hematopoiesis is a direct descendant of the biologic events that occurred in the first SCID patient.[12]

Related Nonsibling Donors

Because most SCID patients did not have an MLC-nonreactive sibling donor, clinicians began to explore other relatives to see if any potential donors were MLC nonreactive. In a limited number of cases, MLC-nonreactive donors were identified that were successfully used to treat cases of SCID.[2,13] When related donors, who were MLC reactive, were used, patients usually died of acute GVHD, suggesting that MLC nonreactivity (HLA-DR locus identity with modern techniques) was a prerequisite for the successful HSCT of SCID without fatal GVHD. This approach to identifying appropriate donors was subsequently applied to other diseases as well.[14]

The lessons

Differences at single class I alleles do not significantly decrease the overall likelihood of event-free survival, whereas class II differences are almost uniformly associated with poor outcome. Thus, the results from the early transplants for SCID were the basis for focusing on identifying donors who were MLC nonreactive or Class II identical.

Unrelated Donors

Because the majority of SCID patients did not have an MLC-nonreactive related donor, the possibility that an MLC-nonreactive unrelated donor might exist who could be a successful donor was explored. Despite the fact that formal programs to identify unrelated MLC nonreactive donors did not exist, a SCID patient, who had a prevalent haplotype, received 7 transplants from an unrelated individual who was MLC nonreactive.[3] The donor and recipient were HLA-B identical but disparate at one HLA-A antigen. The patient was homozygous for HLA-A1 while the donor was heterozygous (HLA-A1, HLA-A2). At 5 months of age the patient received 10×10^6 bone marrow cells/kg by the intravenous route. The bone marrow had been shipped from Denmark to the United States. Ten days later the patient developed a macular rash consistent with GVHD, and PHA-responsive lymphocytes were detected. Three weeks later the patient received a second infusion of 10×10^6 cells. The patient developed detectable lymph nodes and increasingly severe acute GVHD. At 2 months the circulating donor lymphocytes disappeared, and the patient received a third transplant of 17×10^6 cells by the intravenous route. Again the patient developed PHA-responsive donor lymphocytes that persisted for 4 months. A fourth transplant at 13 months of age was performed with 10×10^6 bone marrow cells given intravenously. Again there was an increase in PHA-responsive lymphocytes of donor origin, but by 6 months after HSCT the PHA-responsive donor lymphocytes were no longer detected. Therefore, because of the possibility of hybrid resistance, the patient received 2 doses of cyclophosphamide (25 mg/kg) before HSCT, which consisted of 130×10^6 cells/kg of fresh bone marrow cells. The patient developed PHA-responsive donor lymphocytes and had in vitro responses to both mitogens and antigens. Donor T lymphocytes but no B lymphocytes were present in the patient's circulation. Three months following the fifth transplant, when the patient was about to be discharged from the hospital, he developed severe aplastic anemia with all detectable residual bone marrow cells being of donor origin. Two months later, without preconditioning, the patient received frozen bone marrow cells from his fifth transplant that did not result in any hematopoietic engraftment. Therefore, 4 months later, after preparation with full doses of cyclosphosphamide (50 mg/kg $\times$ 4 days), the patient received 1×10^8 bone marrow cells/kg intravenously. At 2 weeks he developed donor hematopoiesis and acute GVHD. All T lymphocytes were of donor origin. B lymphocytes were detected for the first time, with spontaneous rises in his serum immunoglobulin levels. After discharge, all lymphoid and hematopoietic elements were of donor origin by both karyotyping and cell surface antigen analysis.

The lessons

Previous attempts to use unrelated bone marrow to treat aplastic anemia had been unsuccessful. This patient demonstrated that significant pretransplant immunosuppression may be necessary, even in patients with SCID, to achieve successful donor hematopoietic engraftment. The successful treatment of this patient and other SCID patients with unrelated HSCT were a major impetus for the establishment both of the National Donor Marrow Program and the international cooperation that is now available for obtaining unrelated bone marrow, mobilized peripheral blood cells, and cord blood.

Fetal Liver Cells

Based on studies from neonatally thymectomized mice, it was determined that histoincompatible HSCT could be done if the HSC inoculum was devoid of T lymphocytes capable of causing acute GVHD.[15] Clinical investigators, therefore, attempted to identify sources of human HSC that did not contain T lymphocytes. Their attention initially focused on the potential use of fetal liver, which before 14 to 16 weeks of gestational age is a major source of hematopoiesis in the human fetus. Because no T lymphocytes are found in the circulation after 12 weeks of gestation, it was hypothesized that fetal liver obtained from electively aborted fetuses of less than 12 weeks of gestation would not contain significant numbers of T lymphocytes. Therefore, fetal liver cells could be an HSC source devoid of T lymphocytes. HLA typing was not possible before the transplantation of the fetal liver cells. Therefore, questions existed as to whether clinical benefit would be derived from the engraftment of the histoincompatible HSC.[16] Initially, transplants with fetal liver were unsuccessful, possibly due to the use of cryopreserved fetal liver cells in most cases. The first successful immune reconstitution reported using fetal liver cells was achieved in a patient with SCID due to adenosine deaminase (ADA) deficiency.[17] The patient received 25×10^8 fetal liver cells intraperitoneally when the patient was 5 months old. IgM-bearing cells were detected 19 days after transplantation, and an increase in T lymphocytes was seen by 40 days. PHA-responsive cells were present by day 74. The patient developed in vitro proliferative responses to mitogens, specific antigens (candida), and allogeneic lymphocytes. Immunization with φX174 resulted in a low primary IgM response with little IgG production after a repeat immunization. The patient developed appropriate isohemagglutinin antibodies. The patient was taken off replacement immunoglobulin and did well until 1 year of age when he developed nephrotic syndrome, from which he died.

Subsequent SCID patients without ADA deficiency were also transplanted with fetal liver cells. One patient had the correction of his T-lymphocyte immune deficiency after the transplantation of 8.4×8^7 fetal liver cells intraperitoneally at 13 months of age. He developed GVHD, which lasted for 6 weeks, and had the presence of normal numbers of PHA-responsive T lymphocytes by 12 weeks after transplantation. The patient developed a cutaneous response to candida antigen. Serum IgM levels rose to normal levels by 1 year, but he had no detectable IgG, requiring the continued administration of replacement immunoglobulin.[18] However, subsequent series with larger numbers of patients confirmed the potential of fetal liver cells ± fetal thymus to correct T-lympho-cyte and sometimes B-lymphocyte immunodeficiencies, but also demonstrated that durable engraftment was less than 30% with a low probably of achieving long-term immune reconstitution.

The lessons

The recipients of fetal liver cells demonstrated that fetal liver cells devoid of T lympho-cytes were capable of supporting thymopoiesis without the development of GVHD. The first patient, who developed circulating B lymphocytes, had ADA deficiency. It is now known that cross-feeding can correct ADA deficiency. The investigators could not determine the origin of the circulating B lymphocytes, but they were most likely of recipient origin, while the donor-derived T lymphocytes were the source of ADA. Successful treatment of the ADA-deficient form of SCID with either exogenous enzyme therapy or HSCT results initially in increases in the number of B lymphocytes of recipient origin. Decreased primary and secondary response to φX174 stimulation suggests that there was a lack of normal T- and B-lymphocyte cooperation.

None of the initial recipients of fetal liver cells received any pretransplant chemo-therapy.[19,20] Therefore, it is unlikely that HSC engraftment occurred. The cells that gave rise to T lymphocytes of donor origin may thus have been derived from committed lymphoid progenitors (CLP) that were able to migrate to the recipient thymus, induce its differentiation, and differentiate into circulating T lymphocytes of donor origin.[21] The follow-up of the fetal liver recipients should provide important bio-logic information about the longevity and the breadth of T-lymphocyte immunity derived from CLP.

T-Lymphocyte Depleted HSCT

In 1975 it was first demonstrated in mice that T-lymphocyte depletion of histoincom-patible HSC permitted both the hematological and immunologic reconstitution of irra-diated mice without GVHD.[22] Attempts were therefore undertaken in humans to eliminate T lymphocytes from histoincompatible bone marrow using a variety of tech-niques, both physical and biological. The selective separation of T lymphocytes from HSC by albumin density gradients as well as the suicide of donor T lymphocytes after stimulation by recipient antigens were attempted. None of these approaches led to the correction of the immune deficiency of any SCID patients. Most patients had no signs of the engraftment of any donor cells.

The approach to T-lymphocyte depletion that was first shown to be clinically successful was the physical removal of T lymphocytes based on their agglutination with soybean agglutinin (SBA) followed by the physical rosetting of the residual T lymphocytes by sheep red blood cells (E), which had initially been used to immuno-phenotypically detect T lymphocytes. The combination of SBA agglutination followed by E rosette formation permitted the physical removal of the majority of T lymphocytes from human bone marrow, which could then be used for HSCT. Following preclinical studies in monkeys, patients were treated with HLA haploidentical disparate bone marrow depleted of T lymphocytes.[4,23]

Of the first 6 SCID patients treated with T-lymphocyte depleted MLC-reactive paternal marrow, 5 had durable immune reconstitution, whereas GVHD was limited or nondetectable. None of the patients had chemotherapy before their engraftment. One patient had graft rejection and was successfully retransplanted after pretransplant chemotherapy.

The lessons

The clinical experience confirms the experiments in mice that T-lymphocyte depletion before HSCT could permit the engraftment of histoincompatible HSC without the development of clinically significant or fatal acute GVHD. However, pretransplant immunosuppression is required in some cases to achieve donor immune reconstitution due to the presence of either engrafted maternal T lymphocytes or hybrid resistance. The use of T-lymphocyte depleted HSCT is now in general use for both related and unrelated HSCT.[24]

In Utero HSC Transplantation

A variety of genetic diseases (β- and α-thalassemia, adrenoleukodystrophy, Hurler disease, and so forth) can be cured or stabilized by the postnatal engraftment of normal allogeneic HSC. Some genetic diseases, however, have significant morbidity at the time of birth, suggesting that the engraftment of normal HSC before birth might provide clinical benefit to the patients. Fetuses with hemoglobinopathies have been transplanted in utero with HSC from either fetal liver or T-lymphocyte depleted parental bone marrow without any evidence of sustained hematopoietic engraftment.[25] However, the transplants were performed in fetuses of more than 16 weeks of gestation, by which time the fetuses had T lymphocytes capable of responding to allogeneic cells.[26]

In contrast, 2 SCID patients have been reported who were successfully transplanted with T-lymphocyte depleted parental histoincompatible bone marrow cells.[27,28] In both cases, the genetic basis for the patients' disease was defects in the common γ-chain. The first patient received a total of 18.6×10^6 cells intraperitoneally in 3 injections starting at 16 weeks of gestation. The second patient received 18×10^6 nucleated cells in 2 intraperitoneal injections beginning at 21 weeks of gestation. The clinical outcomes of both patients were similar. Both had PHA-responsive T lymphocytes of donor origin while their B lymphocytes continued to be of recipient origin. In the first case, immunizations were successful with the production of specific antibodies, whereas no information is available about antibody production in the second case. Thus, these patients with the X-linked form of SCID, who have defective natural killer (NK) cells, were able to be successfully engrafted with haploidentical T-cell depleted HSC without the development of any detectable GVHD.

The lessons

In contrast to the SCID patients, the patients with hemoglobinapathies, who have normal immune systems, were not able to be successfully transplanted with haploidentical T-lymphocyte depleted HSC even as early as 16 to 20 weeks of gestation. It is not clear as to whether the immune reconstitution that occurred in the SCID patients was due to HSC engraftment or whether the T lymphocytes are derived from CLP in the HSC inoculum. Nevertheless, the persistence of the donor lymphoid cells was achieved in the SCID patients. Sustained donor lymphoid or hematopoietic engraftment was not achieved in patients with nonimmune genetic diseases, although one patient may have died of in utero GVHD.[29] Both successfully treated SCID patients had X-linked SCID and, therefore, an absence of functional NK cells and the ability to exhibit hybrid resistance. It would be interesting to know if patients with other forms of SCID, who had normal NK function after birth, could be successfully engrafted in utero.

Genetically Corrected HSC

The identification of the molecular basis of most forms of SCID (common γ-chain deficiency, ADA deficiency, interleukin [IL]-7 receptor deficiency, and so forth) made SCID patients logical candidates for the use of genetically corrected autologous HSC. Murine studies had demonstrated that retroviral vectors could transduce pluripotent hematopoietic stem cells as well as committed lymphoid progenitors. Thus, clinical investigators thought that transplantation of genetically corrected autologous HSC could provide all of the benefits associated with the transplantation of allogeneic HSC without the risks of acute or chronic GVHD.

The first gene to be cloned that was associated with SCID was ADA. Researchers in preclinical studies demonstrated that retroviral vectors containing the human ADA gene could transduce both murine HSC and human mature T lymphocytes.[30] The transduction of mature T lymphocytes normalized their intracellular metabolism, demonstrating that the transduced ADA gene produced adequate levels of functioning enzyme. The first human gene transfer trial was in patients with ADA-deficient SCID, who received their own T lymphocytes that had been transduced in vitro.[31] The patients had had adequate numbers of T lymphocytes for the transduction because they were on enzyme replacement therapy. The patients received multiple infusions of the transduced T lymphocytes. The persistence of the transduced cells could be detected for at least 7 years. It was difficult, however, to determine whether any clinical efficacy was associated with the transduced cells because the patients continued on their exogenous enzyme replacement therapy. However, no toxic effects were assessed with the infusion of the transduced T lymphocytes.

Additional patients were then transplanted with a mixture of transduced bone marrow plus transduced peripheral blood. Different retroviral vectors were used for the 2 transductions so that it would be possible to determine the source of any circulating T lymphocytes.[5] Posttransplant analysis of myeloid cells revealed that all transduced cells contain the vector used to transduce bone marrow cells, whereas all the T lymphocytes early after transplantation were derived from the infused mature T lymphocytes. Over the course of the first year the proportion of T lymphocytes derived from the transduced T lymphocytes decreased, whereas the proportion derived from the transduced bone marrow increased, so that by 1 year all the transduced T lymphocytes contained the bone marrow vector. After the patients had their ADA replacement enzyme therapy discontinued, the frequency of their transduced T lymphocytes was 5% and of the bone marrow precursors 25%. Thus, the patients were able to have significant immune reconstitution following the transplantation of the gene corrected cells with the production of specific antibody and the generation of responses to mitogen stimulation. However, the majority of their immune function was due to nontransduced cells, demonstrating the effect of cross-correction between the transduced and the nontransduced cells.

With the identification of defects in the common γ-chain as the basis for the X-link form of SCID, preclinical research was undertaken to evaluate gene transfer. Using a retroviral vector, French investigators transplanted patients with autologous bone marrow transduced with a retroviral vector containing the human common γ-chain gene. In the majority of patients there was the rapid development of T lymphocytes containing the transduced gene as well as the ability to develop antigen-specific T-lymphocyte proliferation and the production of specific antibodies, so that patients could be removed from immunoglobulin therapy.[32] In comparison with the results with the ADA gene transfer, all of the circulating T lymphocytes contained the transduced gene. Unfortunately, 5 patients have developed acute T-lymphocyte leukemia due to the activation of the *LMO2* gene by the inserted gene.[33] The development of leukemia has resulted in gene transfer trials for X-linked SCID being put on hold.

Because of the limited number of transduced T lymphocytes seen in the patients with ADA deficiency, Italian investigators explored the possibility of pretransplant myeloablative therapy to reduce the number of recipient HSC at the time of transplantation. Patients with ADA deficiency transplanted after reduced doses of busulfan have improved immune reconstitution compared with those with no pretransplant chemotherapy, with a larger percentage of both the myeloid cells and T lymphocytes containing the transduced gene.[34] No cases of leukemia have been seen in the patients receiving gene transfer for ADA deficiency.

The lessons

The major difference between the ADA deficiency and X-linked SCID is that a selective advantage exists in vivo for the transduced T lymphocytes in patients with X-linked SCID, whereas no significant selective advantage for the transduced T lymphocytes exists in patients with ADA deficiency due to the cross-correction of nontransduced T lymphocytes by enzyme replacement or enzyme produced by the transduced cells. Therefore, to increase the frequency of the engraftment of the transduced HSC it was necessary to administer pretransplant myelosuppressive therapy with anti-HSC activity. The use of pretransplant myelosuppressive therapy has the associated risks of neutropenia and thrombocytopenia as well as the possibility of the later development of leukemia. Nevertheless, the use of pretransplant myelosuppressive therapy has resulted in an increased frequency of engraftment of the transduced HSC as well as an increase in the frequency of transduced T lymphocytes. The use of pretransplant myelosuppressive therapy is therefore being entertained for gene transfer trials in which the transduced cells will not have a significant selective advantage, including the hemoglobinopathies.

BIOLOGIC INSIGHTS
HSC Niche

Most patients transplanted for SCID with allogeneic HSC, who did not receive pretransplant myelosuppressive therapy, did not have any evidence of sustained donor hematopoiesis as measured by the presence of donor-specific erythroid antigens or donor-specific HLA antigens on myeloid cells. However, when recipient hematopoiesis is eliminated by either severe GVHD or the administration of pretransplant chemotherapy, donor hematopoiesis was readily achieved after HSCT. Although rare donor-derived CD34+ and myeloid cells have been identified in the marrow of SCID patients after transplantation without pretransplant chemotherapy, the exact biologic nature of the cells is not clear. The absence of the sustained production of mature donor erythroid or myeloid elements indicates that clinically significant donor HSC engraftment cannot occur without the creation of "space." The development of bone marrow aplasia due to GVHD after their successful first transplant indicated that donor HSC engraftment had not occurred in the SCID patient.[8]

The complete correction of patients with Wiskott-Aldrich syndrome occurred only after they had received pretransplant myeloablative therapy in addition to immunosuppressive therapy. The first patient transplanted for Wiskott-Aldrich syndrome had improvement only of his lymphoid function with no correction of his platelet abnormalities after having received only immunosuppressive therapy.[35] Thus, the infusion of allogeneic HSC without HSC-targeted myelosuppression to create marrow space has not resulted in donor HSC engraftment.

Induction of Thymopoiesis

Patients with most forms of SCID are characterized by a thymus that maintains the normal architecture seen in fetuses of less than 12 weeks of gestational age. The fetal thymus is characterized by primarily epithelial elements, small blood vessels, no lymphoid elements and, rarely, Hassel corpuscles. The persistence of the fetal architecture indicates that the migration of prethymic lymphoid cells to the thymus is necessary for the induction of thymic differentiation. In a limited number of cases, patients who have been successfully transplanted have had thymus biopsies done, or have been analyzed at autopsy and have shown the development of normal thymic architecture, including normal lymphoid elements, indicating the inductive influence of the lymphoid precursors.

The fetal thymus first contains lymphoid cells at 12 weeks of gestation, which is 4 to 6 weeks after the development of hematopoiesis in the fetal liver. The transplantation of T-lymphocyte depleted HSC in SCID patients is reproductively characterized by the development of circulating immunophenotypic T lymphocytes 3 months after transplantation,[36] suggesting that it takes the CLP and other HSC-derived cells 3 months to develop into prethymic cells, which can then migrate to the thymus, induce thymic differentiation, and generate mature T lymphocytes. These results in SCID patients indicate that any mature T lymphocytes seen in the peripheral blood of HSCT recipients earlier than 3 months after HSCT are due to the homeostatic expansion of the mature T lymphocytes present in the HSC inoculum rather than thymopoiesis.

Duration of the Immune Correction in SCID Patients

An area of ongoing controversy is the duration of the correction of the immune deficiency of patients with SCID following HSCT. Although some SCID patients have functional B lymphocytes, all forms of SCID are characterized by the absence of functional antigen-specific T lymphocytes. Antigen-specific T-lymphocyte function after successful HSCT is due to donor-derived T lymphocytes. When unmodified HSC is used for transplantation, the initial donor-derived T lymphocytes are derived from the mature lymphocytes contained in the HSC inoculum. Starting 3 months after transplantation there is an increasing contribution from thymopoiesis. It is possible to quantitate recipient thymopoiesis by T-cell receptor excision circles (TREC) analysis as well as the immunophenotypic characteristics of naïve recent thymic emigrant (CD4+, CD45RA+) cells. Patients successfully transplanted with T-lymphocyte depleted HSC have the development of T lymphocytes between 3 and 6 months after HSCT. Recipient thymopoiesis peaks 1 year after transplantation.[37] Differences may then occur between patients who have received pretransplant myelosuppression and those who did not receive chemotherapy. Patients who did not receive pre-HSCT chemotherapy and who do not have detectable HSC engraftment have a slow decrease in their thymopoiesis, with a resultant decrease in TREC-positive T lymphocytes and PHA stimulation, as might be expected if the number of CLP capable of entering the thymus decreased due to their lack of self-renewal. Patients who receive chemotherapy and have HSC engraftment have the ongoing production of new CLP capable of supporting recipient thymopoiesis, and the ongoing production of new T lymphocytes. It will be interesting to compare these 2 groups for the persistence of antigen-specific T-lymphocyte responses to infectious antigens, particularly herpes papilloma virus (HPV), because there has been an increased incidence of HPV infections in the long-term recipients who did not receive pretransplant chemotherapy.[38]

Maternal T-Lymphocyte Chimerism

Many SCID patients, especially those with X-linked SCID, are born with circulating T lymphocytes of maternal origin. Rarely do patients have clinical acute GVHD. Some defects in maternal T-lymphocyte function have been identified, including the inability to respond to allogeneic cells.[39] Nevertheless, the presence of maternal T lymphocytes without the presence of acute GVHD raises questions as to the mechanism of the tolerance that had been generated.

Mechanism of Tolerance

The successful HSCT of SCID patients with histoincompatible HSC, either haploidentical parents or incompatible fetal liver, demonstrated that successful HSC engraftment can occur without fatal GVHD. Studies of the successful recipients have revealed several mechanisms of tolerance, including clonal deletion and the presence of IL-10 producing regulatory T lymphocytes.[40,41]

HLA Restriction of Antigen-specific T-Lymphocyte Function

When the first successful fetal liver transplants were performed, Zinkernagel predicted that the recipients of the histoincompatible HSC would fail to achieve the functional reconstitution of T-lymphocyte immunity and would continue to have opportunistic infections because the histoincompatibility between the fetal liver cells and the recipient thymic epithelial cells would result in a lack of development of HLA-restricted antigen-specific T-lymphocyte function.[16] Surprisingly, the patients successfully transplanted with fetal liver cells did develop antigen-specific T-lymphocyte immunity and did not develop clinical opportunistic infections.[42] Subsequent murine experiments demonstrated that histoincompatible HSC could develop into antigen-specific T lymphocytes, restricting the recipient epithelial cell histocompatibility antigens.

The studies of the emergence of antigen restriction after haploidentical T-lymphocyte depleted transplantation for SCID gave additional insights into the development of major histocompatibility complex antigen restriction of human T-lymphocyte function.[43] The evaluation of antigen-specific T-lymphocyte clones during the first 2 years after HSCT demonstrated that the T-lymphocyte clones were restricted by the recipient HLA antigens. However, with time the antigen specificity broadened, and some T-lymphocyte clones restricted by the disparate parental haplotype were identified, suggesting that the T lymphocytes could also be restricted by the HLA alleles of the disparate donor haplotype. The patient who had received pretransplant myeloablative therapy had myeloid cells of donor origin, suggesting that donor antigen-presenting cells were present in the recipient thymus and controlled the development of T-lymphocyte histocompatibility restriction.

SUMMARY

In addition to being curative therapy, HSCT for SCID patients has provided major insights into the immunobiology of allogeneic HSCT, as well as leading the clinical breakthroughs that have resulted in expanding the pool of potential donors for HSCT for non-SCID diseases.

ACKNOWLEDGMENTS

The authors wish to thank Manuela Alvarez-Wilson for her assistance in the preparation of this article.

REFERENCES

1. Gatti RA, Meeuwissen HJ, Allen HD, et al. Immunological reconstitution of sex-linked lymphopenic immunological deficiency. Lancet 1968;2:1366–9.
2. Copenhagen Study Group of Immunodeficiencies. Bone-marrow transplantation from an HLA-A-nonidentical but mixed-lymphocyte-culture identical donor. Lancet 1973;2:1146–50.
3. O'Reilly RJ, Dupont B, Pahwa D, et al. Reconstitution in severe combined immunodeficiency by transplantation of marrow from an unrelated donor. N Engl J Med 1977;297:1311–8.
4. Reisner Y, Kapoor N, Kirkpatrick D, et al. Transplantation for SCID with HLA-1, B, D/DR incompatible marrow fractionated by soy bean agglutinin and sheep red blood cells. Blood 1983;61:341–8.
5. Bordignon C, Notarangelo LD, Nobili N, et al. Gene therapy in peripheral blood lymphocytes and bone marrow for ADA-immunodeficient patients. Science 1995;270:470–4.
6. Ford CE, Hamerton JL, Barnes DWH, et al. Cytological identification of radiation chimaeras. Nature 1956;177:452–4.
7. Jammet H, Mathé G, Pendic B, et al. Etude de six cas d'irradiation totale aiguë accidentelle [Study of six cases of accidental total body irradiation]. Rev Fr Etud Clin Biol 1959;4:210–25 [in French].
8. Meuwissen HJ, Gatti RA, Terasaki PI, et al. Treatment of lymphopenic hypogammaglobulinemia and bone-marrow aplasia by transplantation of allogenic marrow. Crucial role of histocompatibility matching. N Engl J Med 1969;281:691–7.
9. Park BH, Biggar WE, Good RA. Paucity of thymus-dependent cells in human marrow. Transplantation 1972;14:284–6.
10. Speck B, Gluckman E, Haak HL, et al. Treatment of aplastic anaemia by antilymphocyte globulin with or without marrow infusion. Clin Haematol 1978;7:611–21.
11. Parkman R, Rappeport J, Geha R, et al. Complete correction of the Wiskott-Aldrich syndrome by allogeneic bone marrow transplantation. N Engl J Med 1978;209:921–7.
12. Maris MB, Niederwieser D, Sandmaier BM, et al. HLA-matched unrelated donor hematopoietic cell transplantation after nonmyeloablative conditioning for patients with hematologic malignancies. Blood 2003;102:2021–30.
13. Vossen JM, de Koning J, van Bekkum DW, et al. Successful treatment of an infant with severe combined immunodeficiency by transplantation of bone marrow cells from an uncle. Clin Exp Immunol 1973;13:9–20.
14. Beatty PG, Clift RA, Mickelson EM, et al. Marrow transplantation from related donors other than HLA-identical siblings. N Engl J Med 1985;313:765–71.
15. Yunis EJ, Good RA, Smith J, et al. Protection of lethally irradiated mice by spleen cells from neonatally thymectomized mice. Proc Natl Acad Sci U S A 1974;71(6):2544–8.
16. Zinkernagel RM. Thymus function and reconstitution of immunodeficiency. N Engl J Med 1978;198:222.
17. Keightley R, Lawton AR, Cooper MD. Successful fetal liver transplantation in a child with severe combined immunodeficiency. Lancet 1975;2:850–3.

18. Buckley RH, Whisnant JK, Schiff RI, et al. Correction of severe combined immunodeficiency by fetal liver cells. N Engl J Med 1976;297:1076–81.
19. O'Reilly RJ, Kapoor N, Kirkpatrick D. Fetal tissue transplants for severe combined immunodeficiency- their limitations and functional potential. In: Seligmann M, Hitzig WH, editors. Primary immunodeficiencies INSERM symposium No. 16. N Holland (Dutch): Elsevier; 1980. p. 419–33.
20. O'Reilly J, Pollack MS, Kapoor N, et al. Fetal liver transplantation in man and animals. In: Gale RP, editor. Recent advances in bone marrow transplantation. UCLA symposia on molecular and cellular biology, vol. 7. New York: Alan R. Liss, Inc; 1983. p. 799.
21. Mebius RE, Miyamoto T, Christensen J, et al. The fetal liver counterpart of adult common lymphoid progenitors gives rise to all lymphoid lineages, CD45+CD4+CD3– cells, as well as macrophages. J Immunol 2001;166: 6593–601.
22. Boehmer H, Sprent J, Nabholz M. Tolerance to histocompatibility determinants in tetraparental bone marrow chimeras. J Exp Med 1975;141(2):322–34.
23. Reisner Y, Kapoor N, Kirkpatrick D, et al. Transplantation for acute leukemia with HLA-A and -B nonidentical parental marrow cells fractionated with soybean agglutinin and sheep red cells. Lancet 1981;2:327–31.
24. Papadopoulos EB, Carabasi MH, Castro-Malaspina H, et al. T-cell-depleted allogeneic bone marrow transplantation as postremission therapy for acute myelogenous leukemia: freedom from relapse in the absence of graft-versus-host disease. Blood 1998;91:1083–90.
25. Flake AW, Zanjani ED. In utero transplantation for thalassemia. Ann N Y Acad Sci 1998;850:300–11.
26. Carr MC, Stites DP, Fudenberg HH. Dissociation of responses to phytohaemagglutinin and adult allogeneic lymphocytes in human foetal lymphoid tissues. Nature New Biol 1973;241(113):279–81.
27. Flake AW, Roncarolo M-G, Puck JM, et al. Treatment of X-linked severe combined immunodeficiency by in utero transplantation of paternal bone marrow. N Engl J Med 1996;335:1806–10.
28. Wengler GS, Lanfranchi A, Frusca T, et al. In-utero transplantation of parental CD34 haematopoietic progenitor cells in a patient with X-linked severe combined immunodeficiency (SCIDXI). Lancet 1996;348:1484–8.
29. Bambach BJ, Moser HW, Blakemore K, et al. Engraftment following in utero bone marrow transplantation for globoid cell leukodystrophy. Bone Marrow Transplant 1997;19:399–402.
30. Kantoff PW, Kohn DB, Mitsuya H, et al. Correction of adenosine deaminase deficiency in cultured human T and B cells by retrovirus-mediated gene transfer. Proc Natl Acad Sci U S A 1986;83:6563–7.
31. Blaese RM, Culver KW, Miller AD, et al. T lymphocyte-directed gene therapy for ADA-SCID: initial trial results after 4 years. Science 1995;270:475–80.
32. Hacein-Bey-Abina S, Le Deist F, Carlier F, et al. Sustained correction of X-linked severe combined immunodeficiency by ex vivo gene therapy. N Engl J Med 2002;346:1185–93.
33. Hacein-Bey-Abina S, von Kalle C, Schmidt M, et al. A serious adverse event after successful gene therapy for X-linked severe combined immunodeficiency. N Engl J Med 2003;348:255–6.
34. Aiuti A, Slavin S, Aker M, et al. Correction of ADA-SCID by stem cell gene therapy combined with nonmyeloablative conditioning. Science 2002;296: 2410–3.

35. Bach FH, Alberini RJ, Anderson JL, et al. Bone marrow transplantation in a patient with the Wiskott-Aldrich syndrome. Lancet 1968;2:1364–6.

36. O'Reilly RJ, Keever CA, Small TN, et al. The use of HLA non-identical T-cell depleted marrow transplants for correction of severe combined immunodeficiency. Immunodefic Rev 1989;1:273–309.

37. Patel DD, Gooding ME, Parrott RE, et al. Thymic function after hematopoietic stem-cell transplantation for the treatment of severe combined immunodeficiency. N Engl J Med 2000;342:1325–32.

38. Neven B, Leroy S, Decaluwe H, et al. Long-term outcome after hematopoietic stem cell transplantation of a single-center cohort of 90 patients with severe combined immunodeficiency. Blood 2009;113:4114–24.

39. Pollack MS, Kirkpatrick D, Kapoor N, et al. Identification by HLA typing of intrauterine-derived maternal immunodeficiency. N Engl J Med 1982;307:662–6.

40. Rosenkrantz K, Keever C, Bhimani K, et al. Both ongoing suppression and clonal elimination contribute to graft-host tolerance after transplantation of HLA mismatched T cell-depleted marrow for severe combined immunodeficiency. J Immunol 1990;144:1721–8.

41. Bacchetta R, Bigler M, Touraine JL, et al. High levels of interleukin 10 production in vivo are associated with tolerance in SCID patients transplanted with HLA mismatched hematopoietic stem cells. J Exp Med 1994;179:493–502.

42. Roncarolo MG, Yssel H, Touraine JL, et al. Antigen recognition by MHC-incompatible cells of a human mismatched chimera. J Exp Med 1988;168(6):2139–52.

43. Geha RS, Rosen FS. The evolution of MHC restrictions in antigen recognition by T cells in a haploidentical bone marrow transplant recipient. J Immunol 1989;143: 84–8.

HLA-haploidentical Donor Transplantation in Severe Combined Immunodeficiency

Wilhelm Friedrich, MD*, Manfred Hönig, MD

KEYWORDS

- Hematopoietic cell transplantation • HLA-haploidentical
- Severe combined immunodeficiency

Treatment of severe combined immunodeficiency (SCID) by hematopoietic cell transplantation (HCT) changed profoundly in the early eighties when Reisner and colleagues[1] developed a procedure to efficiently reduce the number of T cells contained in marrow grafts responsible for graft-versus-host disease (GVHD), opening the possibility to prevent this complication after HLA-mismatched donor transplantation. The procedure used soybean agglutination in combination with sheep red blood cell rosette formation to fractionate bone marrow cells and provided precursor cell–enriched grafts with drastically reduced T-cell numbers. Reisner and colleagues[2] and, subsequently, several other groups[3–9] were able to demonstrate the potential of T-cell–depleted, HLA-haploidentical parental donor transplants to establish stable immunologic reconstitution in SCID patients with significantly reduced risk for acute and chronic GVHD. Newly developed donor T cells were found to be tolerant to cells of the HLA-haploidentical recipient. Other subsequently developed technologies for T-cell depletion of marrow grafts took advantage of lymphocyte-specific monoclonal antibodies, and more recently, antibodies directed at CD34$^+$ are used to purify CD34$^-$ expressing hematopoietic progenitor cells by positive selection from peripheral blood after their mobilization by granulocyte colony-stimulating factor (GCSF). In patients with SCID, for whom HCT represented the only available curative therapy, these advances led to profound changes in the prognosis of this otherwise lethal disorder, which became uniformly treatable regardless of the availability of a matched family donor. Over the last years, HCT from unrelated matched donors also has been markedly advanced, and both approaches now are well established in the treatment of the disorder. In this review, several pertinent findings in SCID patients undergoing HLA-haploidentical HCT are discussed, and several unresolved issues, such as the

Department of Pediatrics, University of Ulm, Eythstrasse 24, 89075 Ulm, Germany
* Corresponding author. Universitäts-Kinderklinik, Eythstrasse 24, 89075 Ulm, Germany.
E-mail address: wilhelm.friedrich@uniklinik-ulm.de (W. Friedrich).

Immunol Allergy Clin N Am 30 (2010) 31–44
doi:10.1016/j.iac.2009.11.004   immunology.theclinics.com
0889-8561/10/$ – see front matter © 2010 Elsevier Inc. All rights reserved.

nonuniformity of B-cell reconstitution, graft resistance, the role of conditioning, and long-term immune reconstitution, are addressed.

SPECIFIC ASPECTS OF HCT IN SCID

In contrast to other disorders, the profound immunodeficiency in SCID minimizes the risk of immunologic graft rejection, conceptually eliminating the need for immuno-suppressive conditioning before transplantation. This approach of transplanting SCID patients without conditioning, providing a significant advantage because of the reduced toxicity of the procedure, has been widely explored in HLA-identical and HLA-nonidentical transplantation. Because the recipient's hematopoietic system remains intact, there is no advantage for donor precursor cells to engraft and to replace this system, and indeed, evidence for sustained or substantial marrow engraftment by donor cells is usually lacking.[10–13] Nevertheless, lymphocytes of donor origin develop, in contrast to other blood cells, which remain of recipient origin. The potential of HCT to induce stable immune reconstitution in the absence of marrow engraftment raises the obvious question regarding the underlying mechanisms of lymphocyte development in the absence of progenitor cell engraftment in the marrow.

DIFFERENT OUTCOMES AFTER HLA-IDENTICAL AND HAPLOIDENTICAL HCT WITHOUT CONDITIONING

The outcome of HCT in SCID when performed without conditioning differs substan-tially depending on whether nonmanipulated grafts from HLA-identical donors or manipulated, T-cell depleted grafts from HLA-nonidentical donors are used. Mature donor T cells contained in the graft have the capacity to undergo marked proliferation and expansion in the recipient, giving rise to an initial wave of T cells early after trans-plantation. These T cells are responsible for induction of GVHD but also are potentially beneficial and protective, in particular if GVHD is limited or absent, as is commonly the case in SCID patients after sibling transplantation. The scenario obviously is different after HLA-haploidentical transplantation, where this effect of expanding mature T cells is abolished. Development of T cells after T-cell depleted transplantation depends solely on de novo maturation in the thymus. This maturation process is slow. Newly differentiated T cells appear in the circulation only several months after transplanta-tion. In contrast to early developing T cells, which carry predominantly a memory phenotype, newly differentiated T cells disclose a naive phenotype and are rich in a cell marker, the so called T-cell receptor excision circle (TREC), which indicates their recent thymus emigration.[14] These cells are furthermore characterized by a diverse receptor repertoire, in contrast to the more skewed repertoire of early T cells arising by expansion.[15,16] Simultaneously with the delayed development of naive T cells, the previously small thymus characteristic for SCID enlarges in size, as easily visual-ized by ultrasonography.[17] Notably, after transplantation of unmanipulated grafts, a similar kinetics of slow development of naive T cells is observed.[17] It is also inter-esting that T-cell development is similarly delayed in other congenital disorders after HLA-haploidentical, T-cell depleted transplantation, such as infantile osteopetrosis and Wiskott-Aldrich syndrome.[18,19] Furthermore, in SCID patients receiving cytore-ductive conditioning before transplantation for reasons that are discussed in more detail later in the article, the kinetics of slow T-cell reconstitution is not altered.[17] The distinct pattern of T-cell reconstitution after HLA-identical and after HLA-haploi-dentical, T-cell–depleted transplantation is demonstrated in **Fig. 1**.

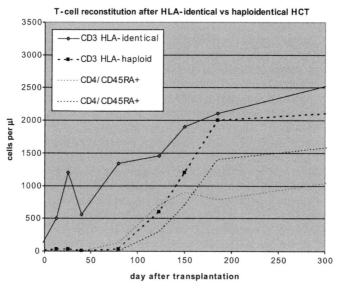

Fig. 1. Different kinetics of development of CD3⁺, but not of naive CD4/CD45RA⁺ T cells after HLA-identical sibling transplantation and HLA-haploidentical, T-cell–depleted transplantation in 2 SCID patients.

Patients remain profoundly immunodeficient for a prolonged period after HLA-haploidentical HCT because it takes up to 4 months until T cells become demonstrable, in contrast to patients after sibling transplantation, in whom early-appearing donor T cells can be effective to control and prevent infections.

Another marked difference after transplantation of grafts with and without T-cell depletion regards reconstitution of humoral immunity. Whereas transplantation of nonmanipulated grafts from HLA-identical donors commonly results in sustained B-cell reconstitution with detection of donor B cells in the circulation, patients after HLA-haploidentical, T-cell–depleted transplantation, when performed without cytoreductive conditioning, commonly fail to develop effective B-cell immunity. With rare exceptions, B cells of donor origin remain absent, as most evident in patients with B− SCID, who fail to develop circulating B cells. In most patients with B+ SCID, autologous B cells persist as expected but fail to become functional, as elegantly shown in a study by White and colleagues.[20] Only exceptionally, such as in patients with IL7R deficiency, CD3 deficiency, and adenosine deaminase (ADA) deficiency, has the functional maturation of autologous B cells after effective T-cell reconstitution been observed. Because in the absence of conditioning, as noted earlier, evidence of substantial engraftment of donor precursor cells in the marrow is usually lacking after both HLA-identical and HLA-nonidentical transplantation, this discrepancy in humoral reconstitution requires an explanation. Graft manipulation and depletion of T cells usually also lead to drastic reduction of B-cell numbers in the grafts. As one possible explanation, it is conceivable that donor B cells arising after HLA-identical transplantation are derived from the pool of donor B cells contained in nonmanipulated grafts. The longevity of mature B cells and their potential to undergo extensive homeostatic proliferation analogous to T cells is well established in murine models and recently also in man,[21,22] and it is conceivable that transfer of mature donor B cells into allogeneic hosts may be effective to establish stable long-term humoral immunity. Nevertheless, the heterogeneity of B-cell reconstitution remains incompletely understood and requires further studies.

Although most patients develop normal and sustained T-cell functions after HLA-haploidentical transplantation without conditioning, a proportion of patients fail to do so, showing either complete graft failures or subnormal T-cell reconstitution. Complete graft failure has been common in particular in ADA deficiency, in SCID patients characterized by the presence of poorly functional T cells, such as in Omenn syndrome, and in SCID patients with functional NK-cell systems. This experience again is in contrast to the outcome after nonmanipulated, HLA-identical sibling transplants, which almost uniformly, regardless of the underlying variant of SCID, will lead to engraftment and development of T-cell immunity. The less-uniform reconstitution after HLA-haploidentical transplantation may be because of several factors restricting T-cell development. One factor may be the absence of an engraftment-facilitating effect mediated by mature donor T cells. Also persistent viral disease, such as cytomegalovirus infections, may suppress lymphoid differentiation and cause poor reconstitution. Furthermore, in certain SCID variants, the environment of the thymus may limit homing of donor precursor cells to specific niches, as has been demonstrated in relevant murine SCID models.[23] The most important factor for subnormal T-cell reconstitution probably is GVHD and its treatment, a complication that may also be induced by maternal T cells secondary to an intrauterine maternofetal transfusion and that may take a subclinical course.[24] Furthermore, graft resistance may be mediated by NK cells, which function in subgroups of SCID patients. Importantly, graft failures can usually be overcome by using pretransplant cytoreductive conditioning. Because this approach also allows marrow engraftment of precursor cells and as a consequence donor B-cell development, conditioning has been used in a significant proportion of patients before initial transplantation.

SURVIVAL AND COMPLICATIONS IN SCID PATIENTS AFTER HLA-HAPLOIDENTICAL HCT

The exploration of HLA-haploidentical HCT in the treatment of SCID has resulted in a series of larger single- and multicenter studies, the latter in particular by groups collaborating in the European Group for Blood and Marrow Transplantation (EBMT) who established the Stem Cell Transplantation for Immunodeficiencies (SCETIDE) registry.[25–29] In the following sections, several issues of HLA-haploidentical HCT are addressed based on these studies, including survival, immune reconstitution, complications, and late outcome.

A multicenter study published in 2003 analyzed the outcome after HCT in patients with primary immunodeficiencies treated in Europe between 1968 and 1999.[25] The study included 475 patients with SCID. Donors in 294 of these cases were HLA-haploidentical parents. The majority (207 cases) had received pretransplant conditioning, consisting mostly of busulfan (8 mg/kg) and cyclophosphamide (200 mg/kg). The 3-year survival rate after HLA-haploidentical transplantation was 54%, which was significantly lower compared with a survival rate of 77% in patients after HLA-identical HCT ($P = .002$) reported in the same study. Importantly, survival rates after haploidentical transplantation have improved significantly over time, from about 50% during the initial period up to 80% during the more recent period, as shown in **Fig. 2**, where survival data of a more recent EBMT survey are demonstrated. It was also noted that the variant of SCID had an impact on survival after HLA-haploidentical HCT, because cases of B− SCID tended to have a poorer prognosis than those of B+ SCID, confirming similar observations in a previous analysis.[29] In the former group,

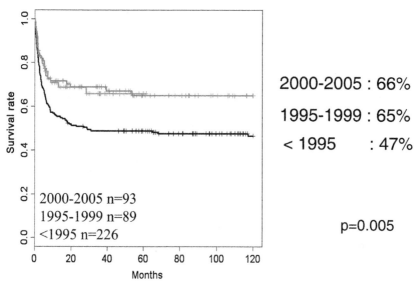

5-year survival after HLA-haploidentical HCT according to time period (EBMT/SCETIDE 2007)

2000-2005 : 66%

1995-1999 : 65%

< 1995   : 47%

2000-2005 n=93
1995-1999 n=89
<1995 n=226

p=0.005

Fig. 2. Survival after HLA-haploidentical HCT in SCID according to year of transplantation. (*Data from* EBMT/SCETIDE registry.)

the use of conditioning before HCT was found to result in better survival, whereas in cases of B+ SCID, survival was not affected by conditioning. For patients with ADA deficiency (n = 26) and for patients with reticular dysgenesis (n = 8), 3-year survival rates were 30%.

In a separate study of 10 patients with reticular dysgenesis, cytoreductive conditioning before HLA-haploidentical HCT was found mandatory to obtain reconstitution of both lymphoid and myeloid functions in this disorder.[30]

Independent predictors of poorer outcome, besides underlying variants of SCID, were the presence of pulmonary infection at transplantation, absence of a protected environment, and occurrence of acute GVHD (grade II or higher). The study also revealed that the incidence of GVHD had decreased over time, from 35% to 40% before 1996 to 22% thereafter (*P*<.001), possibly related to the use of more stringent methods for T-cell depletion, a factor that partly accounted for the observed better survival with time. The main causes of death were infections (56%), GVHD (25%), and B-cell lymphoproliferative syndrome (5%).

In a large single-center study reported by Buckley and colleagues,[27] 77 SCID patients were analyzed after HLA-haploidentical HCT. In this study, a survival rate of 77% was reported, with follow-up after transplantation ranging from 3 months to 16 years. All patients in this study underwent transplants without conditioning. Furthermore, the proportion of patients with B− SCID was very low, in contrast to the European study, in which this proportion was about 35%. An important prognostic factor for survival was noted to be age at transplantation; within the whole group of treated patients, infants who underwent transplant before the age of 3 to 5 months had a survival rate of 95% as compared with a survival rate of 76% in patients beyond that age.

In a previous multicenter EBMT study analyzing prognostic factors for long-term survival, normalization of T-cell immunity at 12 months was identified as a strong favorable indicator, whereas ineffective reconstitution, which may be because of poorly controlled GVHD or other complications, was found to be associated with a substantial mortality.[29]

The basis for improved survival after HLA-haploidentical HCT during more recent periods includes several factors, such as earlier diagnosis resulting in fewer sick patients at the time of transplantation, more effective prevention and treatment of disease-related and transplantation-induced complications (notably infections and GVHD), and effective prevention of graft failure by using conditioning prior to transplantation in patients at risk for this complication.

Efficient prevention of GVHD has been related in particular to the use of highly purified, GCSF-mobilized CD34$^+$ precursor cells from peripheral blood, which are obtainable in high numbers with minimal contamination by T cells.[10] In addition to de novo GVHD caused by imperfect T-cell depletion of grafts, another cause for this complication has been a primary engraftment of transplacentally acquired maternal T cells, which is a common phenomenon in SCID.[24,31] In the study by Buckley and colleagues[27] discussed earlier, 27 of 28 cases with GVHD were noted to have circulating maternal T cells before transplantation. In the authors' own experience of HLA-haploidentical HCT in a cohort of 137 SCID patients, 31 of 59 patients with maternal T-cell engraftment developed GVHD to variable degrees, whereas among the other 78 patients without maternal T cells, only 7 cases developed this complication (Friedrich W, unpublished data, 2009).

HCT WITHOUT AND WITH CONDITIONING

Cytoreductive conditioning in SCID patients, for which most commonly a combination of busulfan and cyclophosphamide is used, has been found to offer several advantages, including, in particular, an improved prevention of graft failure and a high chance of sustained, complete immune reconstitution. In the authors' experience of HLA-haploidentical HCT in SCID, they have observed better overall survival rates in patients who received preparative cytoreductive conditioning compared with those who did not, as demonstrated in **Fig. 3**. Causes of death in the latter group were manifold but included a significant proportion of earlier patients showing complete graft failures. There are, however, obvious disadvantages with this approach, most importantly potentially acute and long-term toxic side effects. In particular, in infants suffering from persistent viral disease or other poorly controllable complications, the risks of conditioning may outweigh its potential benefits. As already mentioned, conditioning does not alter the kinetics of immune reconstitution. Also, the use of highly purified CD34$^+$ cells at comparatively high numbers does not influence the slow pattern of T-cell reconstitution, whether conditioning is used or not.[10] As outlined later in this article, based on studies in long-term surviving patients, some concern has been raised regarding the stability of thymic functions in nonconditioned patients. Nevertheless, the decision to use or not to use conditioning requires careful consideration in each individual case, taking into account potential advantages and disadvantages.

LONG-TERM OUTCOME AND COMPLICATIONS AFTER HLA-HAPLOIDENTICAL HCT

Recently a single-center study analyzing long-term outcome of HCT in a large cohort of SCID patients was reported, assessing the occurrence of clinical events and the quality of life as well as quality and stability of immune functions.[32] Patients were observed from 2 to 34 years (medium 14 years) after transplantation, and the study included 51 cases with HLA-haploidentical donors, 22 cases with matched sibling

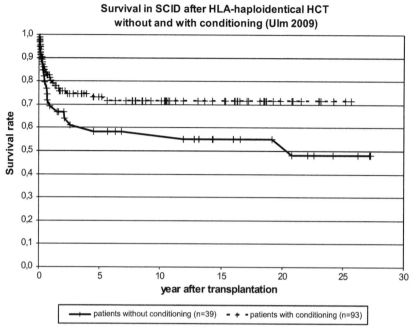

Fig. 3. Overall survival in SCID patients who underwent transplant either without or with preparative cytoreductive conditioning from HLA-haploidentical donors since 1982 at the University of Ulm.

donors, and 15 cases with other HLA-matched family donors. The investigators observed one or more significant late clinical events in about 50% of patients. These included persistent chronic GVHD (in 6 of 51 cases after haploid identical HCT); auto-immune and inflammatory manifestations (in 12 cases within the whole cohort of 90 cases) that included autoimmune hemolytic anemia in 6 cases and chronic inflammatory disease in 3 cases, requiring immunosuppressive treatment over periods of 1.5 to 17 years; opportunistic and nonopportunistic infections, including chronic human papilloma virus (HPV) infections; and prolonged nutritional support. Except HPV infections, these complications were commonly associated with chronic GVHD and its treatment. The rate of infectious complications tended to decrease with increasing time after transplantation, with the exception of severe HPV infection. This infection developed in 23 cases between 4 and 19 years after transplantation and was severe in 9 cases (as defined by the persistence of multiple lesions [>30] for more than 2 years and by poor therapeutic responsiveness) and milder in the others, resolving in 11 of 14 cases. As previously reported by the same group, severe HPV infections were restricted to B+ SCID patients with γc and Jak3 deficiency, leading to the speculation that the continued deficiency in nonlymphoid cells of γc-dependent cytokine signaling, which may play a crucial part in local resistance of keratinocytes, is relevant for the cause of this complication.[33]

An important finding in the study was that T-cell immune reconstitution had failed to normalize in a significant proportion of patients, even after prolonged follow-up. At 1 and 2 years, about 25% of patients had a low CD4 T-cell number, and this percentage remained in the same range at follow-up between 5 and 15 years, confirming previous observations showing that CD4[+] T-cell numbers at 1 and 2 years after HCT were

Table 1
Late immune reconstitution in SCID after HLA-haploidentical HCT (Ulm 2009)

No conditioning

UPN	SCID Variant	Time After BMT (y)	CD3$^+$ Cells/µl	CD4$^+$ Cells/µl	CD8$^+$ Cells/µl	CD4/CD45RA$^+$ Cells/µl	PHA(SI)	Donor B-cell Chimerism	Donor Myeloid Chimerism	IgG Subst
14	B+ (nd)	24	1420	470	820	280	110	No	No	No
15	B+ (γc)	25	1500	650	680	348	540	No	No	Yes
16	B− (Artemis)	26	2150	860	1270	140	140	No	No	Yes
17	B+ (γc)	24	2700	1400	1180	600	290	No	No	Yes
22	B+ (γc)	23	1200	560	430	150	650	No	No	Yes
39	B+ (γc)	17[a]	900	150	863	33	42	No	No	Yes
53	B− (Artemis)	18	1100	840	220	420	470	No	No	Yes
87	B+ (γc)	10[a]	2300	550	1600	30	60	No	No	Yes
88	B+ (γc)	21	1400	600	700	90	120	No	No	Yes
137	B+ (γc)	14	1300	500	610	330	480	Yes	Yes	No
188	B+ (γc)	14	500	140	300	60	115	No	No	Yes
201	B+ (γc)	13	1538	413	844	54	312	No	No	Yes
246	B+ (Jak3)	14	2570	700	1800	200	473	No	No	Yes
247	B+ (Jak3)	14	3600	800	2600	30	120	No	No	Yes
250	B+ (Jak3)	14	1520	1012	418	597	893	No	No	Yes
281	B+ (Jak3)	12	3040	960	1820	633	411	No	No	Yes
282	B− (Artemis)	12	710	520	160	155	140	No	No	Yes

With conditioning

UPN	SCID Variant	Time after BMT (y)	CD3+ Cells/μl	CD4+ Cells/μl	CD8+ Cells /μl	CD4/CD45RA+ Cells/μl	PHA (SI)	Donor B-cell Chimerism	Donor Myeloid Chimerism	IgG Subst
26	ADA	21	2300	570	430	520	550	Yes	Yes	No
36	ADA	19	1470	710	550	380	650	Yes	Yes	No
74	B+ (IL7R)	18	1480	1000	400	390	170	Yes	Yes	No
77	Reticular dysgenesis	17	1930	760	740	400	140	Yes	Yes	No
81	B− (RAG)	21	1200	660	255	323	270	No	No	Yes
84	B+ (γc)	11	1390	562	600	300	690	Yes	Yes	No
101	B+ (Jak3)	17	2160	970	1300	600	260	Yes	Yes	No
128	B− (Artemis)	14	3700	2210	1220	780	760	Yes	Yes	No
172	B+ (γc)	15	2210	1500	490	1190	430	Yes	Yes	No
180	B+ (nd)	15	2170	890	1020	450	430	Yes	Yes	No
197	B− (RAG)	17	1840	1060	680	690	540	Yes	Yes	No
223	B− (RAG)	16	600	400	175	152	349	Yes	Yes	No
241	B+ autosomal	11	500	400	100	16	63	No	No	No
249	B+ (γc)	14	1500	1095	358	613	396	Yes	Yes	No
271	B+ (IL7R)	13	1600	814	682	850	495	Yes	Yes	No
310	B+ autosomal	12	1935	816	956	481	220	Yes	Yes	No

Abbreviations: nd, not determined; PHA, phytohemagglutinin; SI, stimulatory indices; Subst, substitution; UPN, unit patient number.
[a] Both patients died from late complications.

highly predictive of outcome and of late immune T-cell reconstitution.[29] The analysis also revealed that in patients with donor-derived myeloid cells, associated with previous myelosuppressive conditioning, CD4$^+$ T-cell counts tended to be higher at all evaluation times compared with values in patients without donor-derived myeloid cells.

In SCID patients with persisting subnormal reconstitution of T-cell immunity, repeat CD34$^+$ cell infusions without conditioning from the same donors have been attempted to improve graft function. This experience has failed to provide clear evidence for an advantage or efficiency of boost transplants, in particular if given late after initial transplantation.[34]

ADA deficiency is a systemic metabolic disease that may cause other complications beside SCID, including neurologic abnormalities. Late outcome after transplantation was reported in 12 long-term surviving ADA-deficient patients, 6 of whom had undergone HLA-nonidentical transplantation.[35] The analysis revealed that HCT commonly fails to control late central nervous system complications, because 6 of 12 patients showed marked late neurologic abnormalities, including mental retardation, motor dysfunction, and sensorineural hearing deficit. The study failed to reveal a correlation of these abnormalities with the transplant approach used. In another study addressing neurologic outcome in ADA-deficient patients, which included 16 patients and a control group that underwent transplant for nonmetabolic SCID, the authors reported striking behavioral abnormalities in ADA-deficient patients, but, in contrast to the above, no motor function abnormalities.[36]

STABILITY OF T-CELL IMMUNITY AND OF THYMIC FUNCTION

As already discussed, HLA-haploidentical transplantation without conditioning usually results in split chimerism, with donor cell development limited to T cells. Although T-cell lymphopoiesis clearly reflects thymic engraftment of progenitor cells, it remains presently unclear if the thymus is colonized immediately after transplantation during a limited time window when donor precursor progenitor cells are present in the circulation or, alternatively, if transient marrow engraftment takes place, allowing pre–T-cells to emigrate from the marrow to enter the thymus. Because longitudinal studies, with rare exceptions, fail to provide evidence for sustained progenitor cell marrow engraftment, at least based on conventional technologies failing to detect donor cells less than 1%, this latter scenario, in any case, would be operative only temporarily. Based on animal models, a periodical re-colonization of the thymus by precursor cells from the marrow is required to maintain sustained thymopoiesis because stem cells with self-replicating potential are absent in the normal thymus.[37] The possible consequences of the specific situation in SCID patients who undergo transplant without conditioning and in whom periodical re-colonization of the thymus likely does not occur has been addressed in several recent studies that evaluated long-term immune reconstitution and the stability of T-cell lymphopoiesis.[12,13,38,39] In one study,[13] 32 SCID patients surviving longer than 10 years were analyzed (**Table 1**). All patients had received HLA-haploidentical HCT, 17 cases without and 16 cases with myeloablative conditioning. Several findings emerged from this study. Most patients had sustained normal numbers and functions of circulating T cells, including distribution of CD4$^+$ and CD8$^+$ T-cell subsets. In 5 of the 32 patients, however, T cells were decreased to numbers less than 1000 per μl, of whom 3 patients had diminished phytohemagglutinin responses (stimulatory indices <100). Two of the cases with diminished T-cell immunity had died from late complications; 1 from complicating varicella, the other from chronic encephalopathy. Importantly, these 5 patients had never achieved completely normal T-cell immunity after transplantation. There was also a broad range in the number of CD45RA-expressing naive CD4$^+$ cells (see **Table 1**). The number of these cells tended to be lower in patients who underwent transplant without conditioning (mean, 244 per µL; range, 30–600 per µL) in comparison to patients with conditioning (mean, 508 per µL; range, 16–1190 per µL). The only patient in the latter group with a low naive T-cell number had shown only transient myeloid engraftment, similar to 1 other patient, despite conditioning. Patients who underwent transplant without conditioning, with the exception of 1 case, revealed no evidence of myeloid engraftment and lacked donor B-cell engraftment. Lower numbers of naive T cells were associated with diminished total T-cell numbers and/or functions in the 5 patients mentioned earlier, whereas 3 patients with low naive T-cell numbers showed otherwise normal T-cell immunity. Previous determinations of naive T cells in these 3 cases had revealed higher numbers.

Several groups also reported evidence for diminished thymic output in a proportion of long-term surviving SCID patients. In a study by Sarzotti-Kelsoe and colleagues,[38] 10 of 41 patients surviving longer than 10 years after T-cell depleted, haploidentical transplantation without conditioning were noted to lack thymic output of naive T cells, which in this study was based on measurements of TREC as an indicator of recent thymic emigration. Cavazzana-Calvo and colleagues[12] studied 32 SCID patients who survived long-term after transplantation performed either without or with myeloablation. In this study, persistent normal thymopoiesis, as defined by normal proportions of naive CD4$^+$ T cells carrying TREC, was strongly correlated with conditioning and donor myeloid cell engraftment. In nonconditioned patients, sustained thymic function was more common in patients with yc deficiency compared with patients with *RAG* and Artemis deficiency. There was no correlation between thymic function and age at transplantation, and younger age did not provide an advantage with regard to sustained thymic activity. Importantly, the long-term clinical outcome of patients in this study was found not to differ, regardless of the presence or absence of TREC+ T cells.

At present, the relevance of these findings, indicating limited long-term thymopoiesis in a significant proportion of long-term surviving SCID patients, mostly transplanted without myeloablative conditioning and lacking myeloid engraftment, remains open and requires longer observation. Whether the observation of persistent normal thymopoiesis in patients with myeloid chimerism favors the general use of myeloablation before HCT in SCID patients remains to be determined.

SUMMARY

Curative treatment of SCID by HCT remains a challenge, in particular in infants presenting with serious, poorly controllable complications, as is commonly the case in this disorder. In the absence of a matched family donor, HLA-haploidentical transplantation from parental donors represents a uniformly and readily available treatment option, offering a high chance to be successful. Concerning outcomes of HCT in SCID, other important parameters beside survival need to be taken into consideration, in particular, the stability and robustness of the graft and its function as well as potential late complications related either to the disease or to the treatment. At present, strategies in performing haploidentical HCT are not uniform, in particular regarding the indication, intensity, and mode of preparative conditioning. To further advance and to arrive at consistent, solidly founded recommendations, coordinated strategies in the application of the treatment and systematic analysis of outcomes will remain important.

REFERENCES

1. Reisner Y, Kapoor N, Kirckpatrick D, et al. Transplantation for acute leukemia with HLA-A and B nonidentical parental bone marrow fractionated with soybean agglutinin and sheep red blood cells. Lancet 1981;2:327–31.
2. Reisner Y, Kapoor N, Kirkpatrich D, et al. Transplantation for severe combined immunodeficiency with HLA-A, B, D, DR incompatible parental marrow cells fractionated with soybean agglutinin and sheep red blood cells. Blood 1983;61: 341–8.
3. Friedrich W, Goldmann SF, Vetter U, et al. Immunoreconstitution in severe combined immunodeficiency after transplantation of HLA haploidentical, T-cell-depleted bone marrow. Lancet 1984;1(8380):761–4.
4. Friedrich W, Goldmann SF, Ebell W, et al. Severe combined immunodeficiency: treatment by bone marrow transplantation in 15 infants using HLA-haploidentical donors. Eur J Pediatr 1985;144:125–30.
5. Buckley RH, Schiff SE, Sampson HA, et al. Development of immunity in human severe primary T-cell deficiency following haploidentical bone marrow stem cell transplantation. J Immunol 1986;136:2398–407.
6. Cowan MJ, Wara DW, Weintrub PS, et al. Haploidentical bone marrow transplantation for severe combined immunodeficiency disease using soybean agglutinin-negative, T-depleted marrow grafts. J Clin Immunol 1985;5:370–6.
7. Fischer A, Durandy A, De Villarty JP, et al. HLA-haploidentical bone marrow transplantation for severe combined immunodeficiency using E-rosette fractionation and cyclosporine. Blood 1986;67:444–9.
8. Morgan G, Linen DC, Knott LT, et al. Successful haploidentical mismatched bone marrow transplantation in severe combined immunodeficiency: T-cell removal using CAMPATH-1 monoclonal antibody and E-rosetting. Br J Haematol 1986; 62:421–30.
9. O'Reilly RJ, Keever CA, Small TN, et al. The use of HLA-non-identical T-cell-depleted marrow transplants for correction of severe combined immunodeficiency disease. Immunodefic Rev 1989;1:273–309.
10. O'Reilly RJ, Small TN, Friedrich W. Hematopoietic cell transplant for immunodeficiency diseases. In: Thomas ED, Blume KG, Forman SJ, editors. Hematopoietic cell transplantation. 2nd edition. Malden (MA): Blackwell Science; 2004. p. 1430–42.
11. Tjonnfjord GE, Steen R, Veiby OP, et al. Evidence for engraftment of donor-type multipotent CD34+ cells in a patient with selective T-lymphocyte reconstitution after bone marrow transplantation. Blood 1994;84:3584–9.
12. Cavazzana-Calvo M, Carlier F, Le Deist F, et al. Long-term T-cell reconstitution after hematopoietic stem-cell transplantation in primary T-cell–immunodeficient patients is associated with myeloid chimerism and possibly the primary disease phenotype. Blood 2007;109:4576–80.
13. Friedrich W, Hoenig M, Mueller SM, et al. Long-term follow-up in patients with severe combined immunodeficiency treated by bone marrow transplantation. Immunol Res 2007;80:6621–8.
14. Krengler W, Schmidlin H, Cavadini G, et al. On the relevance of TCR rearrangement circles as molecular markers for thymic output during experimental graft-versus-host disease. J Immunol 2004;172:7359–67.
15. Knobloch C, Friedrich W. T cell receptor diversity in severe combined immunodeficiency following HLA-haploidentical bone marrow transplantation. Bone Marrow Transplant 1991;8(5):383–7.

16. Sarzotti M, Patel DD, Li X, et al. T cell repertoire development in humans with SCID after nonablative allogeneic marrow transplantation. J Immunol 2003; 170(5):2711–8.

17. Müller SM, Kohn T, Schulz A, et al. Similar pattern of thymic-dependent T-cell reconstitution in infants with severe combined immunodeficiency after human leukocyte antigen (HLA)-identical and HLA-nonidentical stem cell transplantation. Blood 2000;96(13):4344–9.

18. Schulz AS, Classen CF, Mihatsch WA, et al. HLA-haploidentical blood progenitor cell transplantation in osteopetrosis. Blood 2002;99(9):3458–60.

19. Friedrich W, Schütz C, Schulz A, et al. Results and long-term outcome in 39 patients with Wiskott-Aldrich syndrome transplanted from HLA-matched and mismatched donors. Immunol Res 2009;44(1–3):18–24.

20. White H, Thrasher A, Veys P, et al. Intrinsic defects of B cell function in X-linked severe combined immunodeficiency. Eur J Immunol 2000;30(3):732–7.

21. Cabatingan MS, Schmidt MR, Sen R, et al. Naive B lymphocytes undergo homeostatic proliferation in response to B cell deficit. J Immunol 2002;169(12): 6795–805.

22. van Zelm MC, Szczepanski T, van der Burg M, et al. Replication history of B lymphocytes reveals homeostatic proliferation and extensive antigen-induced B cell expansion. J Exp Med 2007;204(3):645–55.

23. Prockop SE, Petrie H. Regulation of thymus size by competition for stromal niches among early T cell progenitors. J Immunol 2004;173:1604–11.

24. Mueller SM, Ege M, Pottharst A, et al. Transplacentally acquired maternal T lymphocytes in severe combined immunodeficiency: a study of 121 patients. Blood 2001;98(6):1847–51.

25. Antoine C, Muller S, Cant A, et al. Long-term survival after transplantation of haematopoietic stem cells for immunodeficiencies: report of the European experience 1968–1999. Lancet 2003;361:553–60.

26. Bertrand Y, Landais P, Friedrich W, et al. Influence of severe combine immunodeficiency phenotype on the outcome of HLA non-identical, T cell depleted bone marrow transplantation: a retrospective European survey from the European group for bone marrow transplantation and the European society for immunodeficiency. J Pediatr 1999;134:740–8.

27. Buckley RH, Schiff SE, Schiff RI, et al. Hematopoietic stem-cell transplantation for the treatment of severe combined immunodeficiency. N Engl J Med 1999;340: 508–16.

28. Fischer A, Landais P, Friedrich W, et al. European experience of bone marrow transplantation for severe combined immunodeficiency. Lancet 1990;2:850–4.

29. Haddad E, Landais P, Friedrich W, et al. Long-term immune reconstitution and outcome after HLA-nonidentical T-cell-depleted bone marrow transplantation for severe combined immunodeficiency: a European retrospective study of 116 patients. Blood 1998;91:3646–53.

30. Bertrand Y, Mueller SM, Casanova JL, et al. Reticular dysgenesis: HLA nonidentical bone marrow transplants in a series of 10 patients. Bone Marrow Transplant 2002;29(9):759–62.

31. Pollack MS, Kirkpatrick D, Kapoor N, et al. Identification by HLA typing of intrauterine-derived maternal T-cells in four patients with severe combined immunodeficiency. N Engl J Med 1982;307:662–6.

32. Neven B, Leroy S, Decaluwe H, et al. Long-term outcome after hematopoietic stem cell transplantation of a single-center cohort of 90 patients with severe combined immunodeficiency. Blood 2009;113(17):4114–24.

33. Laffort C, Le Deist F, Favre M, et al. Severe cutaneous papillomavirus disease after haemopoietic stem-cell transplantation in patients with severe combined immune deficiency caused by common gamma cytokine receptor subunit or JAK-3 deficiency. Lancet 2004;363(9426):2051.

34. Booth C, Ribeil JA, Audat F, et al. CD34 stem cell top-ups without conditioning after initial haematopoietic stem cell transplantation for correction of incomplete haematopoietic and immunological recovery in severe congenital immunodeficiencies. Br J Haematol 2006;135(4):533-7.

35. Hoenig M, Albert MH, Schulz A, et al. Patients with adenosine deaminase deficiency surviving after hematopoietic stem cell transplantation are at high risk of CNS complications. Blood 2007;109(8):3595-602.

36. Rogers MH, Lwin R, Fairbanks L, et al. Cognitive and behavioral abnormalities in adenosine deaminase deficient severe combined immunodeficiency. J Pediatr 2001;139(1):44-50.

37. Frey JR, Ernst B, Surh CD, et al. Thymus-grafted SCID mice show transient thymopoiesis and limited depletion of V beta 11+ T cells. J Exp Med 1992;175(4):1067-71.

38. Sarzotti-Kelsoe M, Win CM, Parrott RE, et al. Thymic output, T-cell diversity, and T-cell function in long-term human SCID chimeras. Blood 2009;114(7):1445-53.

39. Mazzolari E, Forino C, Guerci S, et al. Long-term immune reconstitution and clinical outcome after stem cell transplantation for severe T-cell immunodeficiency. J Allergy Clin Immunol 2007;120(4):892-9.

Haploidentical Bone Marrow Transplantation in Primary Immune Deficiency: Stem Cell Selection and Manipulation

David Hagin, MD, Yair Reisner, PhD*

KEYWORDS

- Immunodeficiency • Stem cell transplantation
- T cell depletion

Primary immunodeficiency (PID) describes a group of inherited disorders character-ized by impairment of innate or adaptive immunity. Although rare, PID commonly leads to lethal complications mainly as a result of severe and recurrent infections. In the last 50 years there has been enormous progress in understanding and identifying the genetic variability causing PID, with more than 150 different primary immune defi-ciency syndromes known today.[1–3] Despite this variability in etiology, especially for severe cases of immune deficiency, hematopoietic stem cell transplantation (HSCT) remains the major curative treatment to correct the immunodeficiency and reverse the predicted poor prognosis. The first HSCT for treatment of severe combined immu-nodeficiency was performed in 1968 using a bone marrow donation from an human leukocyte antigen (HLA) identical sister to correct the immune function of an infant with severe combined immunodeficiencies (SCID).[4] However, because of the lethal complication of graft versus host disease (GVHD), the procedure could be employed only in patients who had an HLA identical donor.[5] It was 12 years later that successful stem cell selection, using differential agglutination with soybean agglutinin (SBA) and subsequent T cell depletion (TCD) with sheep red blood cells (SRBC), made it possible to perform lifesaving stem cell transplantations using a haploidentical stem cell donor, without causing lethal GVHD.[6]

Department of Immunology, Weizmann Institute of Science, PO Box 26, Rehovot 76100, Israel
* Corresponding author.
E-mail address: yair.reisner@weizmann.ac.il (Y. Reisner).

Immunol Allergy Clin N Am 30 (2010) 45–62
doi:10.1016/j.iac.2009.11.002
0889-8561/10/$ – see front matter © 2010 Elsevier Inc. All rights reserved.

T CELL DEPLETED STEM CELL TRANSPLANTATION

Stem cell transplantation offers a curative treatment for many patients with a severe form of immune deficiency, as well as malignant and nonmalignant hematologic disorders. As an identical, related, stem cell donor is available only in a small minority of cases (15%–20%),[7] alternative donors are needed. The 2 alternative options are allogeneic stem cell transplantation from an unrelated identical donor and haploidentical related donor (in which the donor and recipient share only 1 of 2 possible HLA haplotypes). For the first option, despite the world registry network, the odds of finding a matched unrelated donor in the registries varies with the patient's race and ranges from approximately 60% to 80% for whites to less than 10% for ethnic minorities.[8,9] Another major disadvantage is the time required to identify a donor from a potential panel; the severely immune compromised patient may succumb to severe infectious complications during this time. Furthermore, with the development of molecular analysis, close matching has become more accurate in an attempt to reduce the risk of GVHD but, at the same time, the chance of finding a suitable matched donor reduces even more. For these reasons, allogeneic identical stem cell transplantation is not available for most treatment candidates. On the other hand, virtually all patients have a readily available haploidentical family member. Using a full haplotype mismatched related donor offers several significant advantages:

1. Immediate donor availability
2. Immediate access to donor-derived cellular therapies if required after transplantation, including repeated transplantation from the same donor or from the other haploidentical parental donor in case of graft failure
3. Ability to select the donor of choice out of several available relatives by their clinical status and natural killer (NK) alloreactivity.

However, the use of haploidentical donors has presented a major challenge in the past 4 decades, because of life-threatening GVHD. Following a lead originally attributed to Delta Uphoff,[10] the possibility that fetal liver at the appropriate time in development, lacking post-thymic immunocompetent cells, could be used as a source of stem cells without producing GVHD was studied.[11,12] Later, similar results were achieved using splenocytes from neonatally thymectomized mice to protect lethally irradiated mice without causing GVHD.[11]

Further work in the late 1970s using specific anti-T cell antibodies in mice[10,11] or antilymphocyte antibodies in rats[13] demonstrated that TCD can effectively enable radioprotection without GVHD. Furthermore, as many as 0.3% of mature T cells in the donor graft can cause a high incidence of lethal GVHD.[13] In parallel with this work, we have demonstrated that the lectin SBA can effectively separate hemapoietic stem cells from T cells, to enable successful bone marrow transplantation in lethally irradiated mice from fully disparate donors. This procedure was established based on the earlier observation that the peanut agglutinin (PNA) and SBA, which are exposed on hematopoietic stem cells (HSCs), are masked by sialic acid in the maturation process in the thymus medulla (**Fig. 1**).[14,15]

It was then clear that the key to successful haploidentical stem cell transplantation is dependent on a highly T cell depleted stem cell graft.

Based on the initial work on rodents with SBA[16,17] we further tested our ability to purify bone marrow stem cells from mature T cells in primates. Although a modification of the separation protocol was needed, a successful TCD was achieved[18] and an allogeneic T cell depleted stem cell transplantation was fully engrafted without causing GVHD.[19]

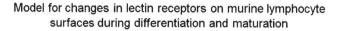

Model for changes in lectin receptors on murine lymphocyte
surfaces during differentiation and maturation

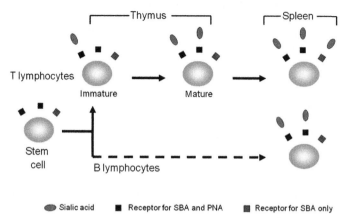

Fig. 1. Sialylation of PNA and SBA receptors during thymic differentiation. (*From* Reisner Y. Changes in lectin receptors during lymphocyte differentiation: application to bone marrow transplantation. Lectins Biol Biochem Clin Biochem 1983;3:681; with permission.)

In 1980, following further adaptation to human bone marrow to attain more than 3 log TCD, this approach finally enabled us to perform an allogeneic haploidentical bone marrow transplantation on a 10-month-old girl with acute leukemia.[6] Eight weeks after transplantation of a haploidentical paternal graft, the girl showed complete recovery of the stem cell graft with T cells and other marrow cells of the donor type, without any evidence of GVHD in the absence of GVHD prophylaxis. In parallel, this method was used successfully in 1980 for the treatment of the first SCID patient with his mother's bone marrow.[20]

The era of T cell depleted stem cell transplantations had begun.

METHODS OF TCD

Three major TCD methods have been used successfully for the treatment of PID patients.

Stem Cells Fractionation by Lectins

Lectins are sugar-binding proteins that are highly specific for their carbohydrate moieties. Stem cell fractionation using lectins is based on the principle that cell subpopulations expressing different lectin receptors can be separated by differential agglutination. Of the different lectins used for cell separation and identification, plant lectin SBA was shown to be useful in the separation of bone marrow cells and depletion of mature T cells.[18] After several modifications, an efficient and rapid technique was developed for the large-scale removal of T lymphocytes from human bone marrow. The method achieved a highly purified cell population rich in blast cells and all myeloid precursors but depleted of T lymphocytes. Briefly, there are 4 main steps in this process[6]: (1) selective removal of red blood cells (RBCs) by gravity sedimentation; (2) agglutination with SBA and differential sedimentation of the agglutinated (SBA+) cells; (3) removal of E-rosette forming T cells from the SBA− cell fraction by centrifugation over Ficoll (RBCs form around human T cells on incubation); (4) repetition of the E-rosetting step using neuraminidase-treated sheep RBCs to eliminate residual T cells in the SBA⁻E⁻ fraction. The cells collected at the end of the process (SBA⁻E⁻E_N⁻) were used for transplantation.

Following the successful transplantation of a haploidentical stem cell graft in a patient with acute leukemia as described earlier,[6] this method was used in the treatment of patients with SCID using a haploidentical stem cell parental graft.[20–22]

Although the initial reports were limited because of the small number of recipients and short duration of follow-up, several significant issues were demonstrated. First, although more than 1 stem cell donation was needed in some of the patients, durable engraftment was achieved. Each of the patients developed mixed chimerism with T cells that were exclusively of donor type, and non-T populations that were either of mixed or host origin. Second, full reconstitution of cell-mediated immunity and partial reconstitution of humoral immunity was achieved. Despite the capability of engrafted paternal lymphocytes for a strong alloreactive response, reactivity against host cells in vitro was diminished. Third, no significant GVHD developed.

A modification of the method described is the use of E-rosetting with neuraminidase-treated SRBCs without prior lectin separation. Although the degree of TCD was less than that described earlier, requiring posttransplant immunosuppressive treatment to prevent GVHD, it was hoped that the presence of more donor T cells in the graft might enable better engraftment and faster immune reconstitution.[23]

TCD Using Anti-T Cells Monoclonal Antibodies

Shortly after the development of lectin-based cell separation, another method using monoclonal antibodies was examined. The first antibody used was the anti-CD3 monoclonal antibody OKT3. Although engraftment was achieved, significant acute GVHD (aGVHD) could not be prevented.[24,25] This could be explained by insufficient ex vivo TCD and by the inability of this murine antibody to activate human complement and continuously inactivate donor T cells after transplantation.

In 1983 a new monoclonal antibody was presented by Hale and colleagues[26] The antibody, a rat monoclonal anti-CD52 designated CAMPATH 1(alemtuzumab in the humanized form), has been proved to fix human complement and efficiently eliminate lymphocytes (>99% depletion) when incubated with complement-containing autologous plasma, while sparing the colony-forming cells in the bone marrow. Comparison between the 2 methods for TCD showed a similar degree of reduction in bone marrow T cells (99.8% for SBA vs 99.4% for Campath 1).[27] Soon after, Campath 1 became widely used for T cell depletion in allogeneic bone marrow transplantation for the treatment of malignant diseases and a significant reduction in the occurrence and degree of GVHD relative to untreated bone marrow was reported, although most of these preliminary studies described patients who received transplants from HLA-matched donors[28–30] and with posttransplant immune suppression. Since then, anti-CD52 antibodies has been used for prevention of graft rejection[31] in organ transplantation and as an antineoplastic drug.[32]

Positive Selection of Hematopoietic CD34+ Stem Cells

In the late 1990s, following a successful positive selection of CD34+ stem cells,[33–35] this approach afforded a third option for TCD. The most commonly used methods, Isolex or the Milteney CliniMACS system, based on magnetic beads attached to an anti-CD34 antibody, enable marked purification of CD34+ stem cells.[36] This procedure can be performed with or without additional negative depletion of CD3+ cells. In particular, in this method peripheral blood can be used as a source of stem cells affording up to 4 log TCD.

The following paragraphs summarize the efficacy of TCD HSCT in relation to overall survival, GVHD prevention, and recovery after transplantation and immune reconstitution. As most of the larger retrospective studies regarding HSCT in PID compare TCD haploidentical HSCT to unmanipulated identical HSCT (either related or unrelated), without distinguishing between the method used for T cell depletion, most of the data presented focuses on the differences between TCD HSCT and unfractionated HSCT. Data regarding the effect of the method used for TCD on posttransplantation outcome is presented where available.

LONG-TERM SURVIVAL AFTER TCD HSCT

A review of the literature regarding the long-term results of T cell depleted stem cell transplantation reveals an unexpected variability in the outcome and survival of patients treated. Some of the disparity could result from the nature of the primary disease but other variables should be considered, such as supportive care, the degree of TCD, pretreatment conditioning regimen (CR) and posttransplantation prophylaxis.

Survival in SCID Patients

When considering the information on the overall survival of TCD HSCT in SCID patients, a careful analysis of the data should be made. Although the overall survival in the European Group for Blood and Marrow Transplantation multicenter study, which was published in 1998, showed a poor prognosis of 52% long-term survival,[37] almost at the same time 2 other studies published by Buckley and colleagues[38] and Small and colleagues[39] in North America reported a long-term survival rate of near 80% (**Fig. 2A**). However, there are some significant differences between the groups. The method used for TCD in the North American studies was SBA and E-rosetting; the depletion in the European study comprised several methods including E-rosetting ± albumin gradient separation, SBA and E-rosetting or monoclonal antibodies with complement lysis. The difference in the degree of TCD might be associated with the disparity presented. In addition, the CR and the posttransplantation prophylactic treatment were different between the groups. In consideration of the marked sensitivity of SCID patients even to mild conditioning, in the early studies during the 1980s the North American groups preferred to avoid using conditioning and largely resorted to repeated transplantation. Moreover, no GVHD prophylaxis was used. On the other hand, in the European study conditioning and posttransplantation prophylaxis were given in 73% and 33% of the cases, respectively. Two other areas of uncertainty are the phenotypical composition of the SCID population involved (as discussed later) and the quality of supportive care used. The quality of supportive care is supported by a more recent analysis from the European group (based on data gathered in the SCE-TIDE (Stem Cell Transplantation for Immunodeficiencies) registry and includes the largest cohort of patients described) demonstrating significant improvement in long-term survival with time (**Fig. 2B**)[40] (reaching near 80% in transplantation performed after 1996, in accordance with the data presented by the North American groups). In 1996, CD34+ positive selection[40] began to be used as a method for TCD. Better TCD and improvement in the diagnosis and treatment of infectious complications can explain improved survival.

There is no doubt that related HLA identical stem cell transplantations result in the highest survival with more than a 90% long-term survival rate.[41] This survival rate can be further improved, even with haploidentical TCD HSCT, when performed in the neonatal period.[42] However, for most patients,[39] the haploidentical stem cell graft is more than a reasonable alternative in the absence of an HLA identical family member,

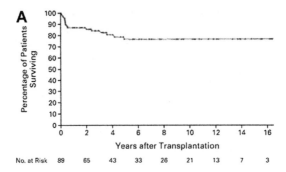

No. at Risk   89   65   43   33   26   21   13   7   3

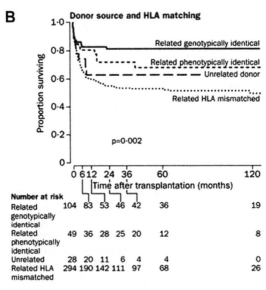

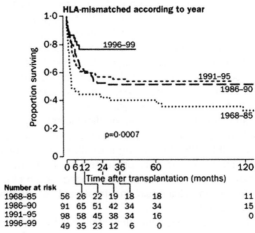

even compared with unmanipulated, matched, unrelated donor graft with ~80% survival rate.[37]

Despite the favorable results of TCD HSCT, there is much diversity in the outcome of SCID patients based on the disease phenotype and genetic cause. To simplify matters, based on the existence of B lymphocytes, SCID can be separated into 2 main groups: the first is the autosomal recessive (AR) inherited, characterized by the absence of T and B lymphocytes but by the presence of normal NK cells (T−B−NK+ SCID); the second is either X-linked or AR, characterized by the absence of T cells and NK cells but by the presence of nonfunctional B cells (T−B+NK− SCID). In general, the results of haploidentical TCD HSCT are significantly better for patients with T−B+NK− SCID (60% survival) than for T−B−NK+ SCID (35%).[43] Although with time, and younger age at transplantation and the use of conditioning treatment, these results improved, the outcome of B− SCID transplantations are still less favorable with overall survival near 50%.[41,43] Similar disparity was not found with an identical related stem cell donor.[40] It is traditionally believed that existing NK cells are responsible for graft rejection, causing a low rate of engraftment and poor prognosis.

ADA SCID represents another group of patients in which the efficacy of TCD HSCT is difficult to evaluate. In a retrospective study, data from 87 patients demonstrated a 1-year survival of 88%, 67%, and 29% to 43% with related identical donor, unrelated identical donor, and haploidentical donor, respectively.[40] However, when evaluating patients who received a highly T cell depleted haploidentical stem cell graft, without any pretransplantation treatment, the long-term survival rate approximates 75%, almost the same as in other B+ SCID.[44]

Survival in Non-SCID PID Patients

Despite supportive management, premature mortality mostly as a result of infectious complications, has led to the use of HSCT as a curative treatment. Although a heterogeneous group of diseases, combined analysis of the available data predicts an unfavorable outcome for TCD haploidentical HSCT compared with matched related HSCT (71% vs 42% 3-year survival),[40] without evidence for improvement over time.

Of the non-SCID PIDs treated with HSCT, patients with Wiskott-Aldrich syndrome (WAS) are the largest group. A recent analysis of 96 patients treated with HSCT for WAS showed inferior results for haploidentical HSCT relative to mostly unmanipulated identical HSCT, either related or unrelated (55%, 88% and 71%, respectively).[45]

The data suggest that when considering the treatment of choice for non-SCID PID, as the threat of imminent death does not exist, a search for a fully matched stem cell donor should be conducted, as long as the procedure is performed at a young age.[46]

Fig. 2. Long-term survival rate after T cell depleted haploidentical SCT. (*A*) Kaplan-Meier survival curve for 89 patients with severe combined immunodeficiency who received stem cell transplants; 12 received transplants from related identical donors. *From* Buckley RH, Schiff SE, Schiff RI, et al. Hematopoietic stem-cell transplantation for the treatment of severe combined immunodeficiency. N Engl J Med 1999;340(7):510; with permission. (*B*) Cumulative probability of survival in SCID patients, according to donor source (related or unrelated donor) and HLA matching, and year of transplantation. (*From* Antoine C, Müller S, Cant A, et al. Long-term survival and transplantation of haemopoietic stem cells for immunodeficiencies: report of the European experience 1968–99. Lancet 2003;361(9357):556; with permission.)

Method of T Cell Depletion and Survival

Because of the lack of data comparing the efficacy of the different methods for TCD, it is almost impossible to conclude which is the preferred method for T cell depletion. One study has demonstrated reduced engraftment and survival in T−B−NK+ SCID patients when monoclonal antibodies were used for T cell depletion.[43] Similarly, although not analyzed for statistical significance, a slightly reduced survival was implicated when comparing the long-term sequelae of anti-CD52 depletion and CD34+ positive selection (19/27 vs 19/22).[36] As these studies reflect separation procedures which, in part, were performed more than 10 years ago, it is more than reasonable to assume that improvement in separation techniques will render this difference insignificant.

GVHD AND TCD HSCT

TCD was developed as a method to prevent GVHD when using haploidentical stem cell grafts. The prevention of GVHD is of great importance as retrospective analysis has shown it is a significant risk factor for reduced survival when appearing either in the early form of aGVHD or when present 6 months after transplantation in the form of cGVHD.[37,40]

In addition, as was recently suggested, GVHD might impair thymic function and affect long-term T cell immune reconstitution.[47,48] Despite the initial results which showed near complete prevention of GVHD, data presented in larger studies describe a higher incidence of GVHD than previously expected. However, the incidence and severity of GVHD was significantly lower than that observed with unmanipulated stem cell grafts.

Acute GVHD

In several studies of SCID patients, different rates of acute GVHD were reported. For TCD haploidentical HSCT the incidence rate was 34% at the Duke University group (grades I–III),[2] and between 40% and 22% in the European group (grade II or higher) with improvement over the years.[40] These results are comparable and somewhat better than those achieved with identical related HSCT (30.8%–40%[2,41]), but significantly superior in incidence and severity compared with patients receiving transplants from unmanipulated, matched, unrelated donor (73.1% incidence, 3/41 patients died as a consequence of aGVHD, the most common cause of death).[41]

No GVHD prophylaxis was used in the Duke series, but patients in the European group who received haploidentical TCD HSCT were treated with at least 2 months of cyclosporin A. Considering the mild degree of the GVHD that developed, and the small reduction (if any) in the incidence of GVHD in patients receiving prophylactic treatment, careful evaluation of the risks of chemoprophylactic treatment should be made, as it is possible that more vigorous T cell depletion by itself would achieve similar results.

Most of the cases of GVHD after haploidentical TCD HSCT occurred when there was persistence of transplacentally transferred maternal T cells,[2] a phenomenon that was seen in up to 40% of SCID patients.[49]

There is general lack of data regarding the prevalence and severity of acute GVHD after HSCT for non-SCID patients. The European study describes aGVHD as a poor prognostic factor independent of the origin of the donor.[40] In a WAS study the incidence of significant aGVHD (grades II–IV) was affected by the origin of the donor with an incidence of 16% for HLA identical sibling donors, 30% for other related donors, and 56% for unrelated donor transplant, although in the last 2 groups, not all of the grafts were T depleted.[46]

Chronic GVHD

In SCID patients chronic GVHD is an infrequent complication. In several series of T cell depleted haploidentical HSCT, there was a low incidence (<2%) of low-grade chronic GVHD (cGVHD).[2,36,41] In a more recent study describing a long-term follow-up of up to 34 years after HSCT, the incidence of cGVHD when using haploidentical HSCT was 10%. At least in some of these patients the disease was of higher grade and disseminated.[50] These frequencies are significantly lower than those described for matched unrelated donors (23%).[41]

Method of TCD and GVHD

It is reasonable to assume that better TCD will result in lower incidence and severity of GVHD; however, in the absence of well-controlled comparative studies, this point cannot be easily demonstrated.

Several issues should be mentioned about GVHD. GVHD should be considered as a double risk for the patient: the clinical risk of severe and lethal disease and the long-term immunologic risk of thymic dysfunction and reduced thymopoiesis. Posttransplantation prophylaxis could be considered as a measure for prevention of GVHD, but the possible risk of thymic damage without an obvious benefit of the preventive treatment as described earlier, requires a careful and thoughtful decision making when choosing the appropriate treatment for the patient.

ENGRAFTMENT AND IMMUNE RECONSTITUTION FOLLOWING TCD HSCT
Engraftment

In the first series of TCD HSCT in SCID patients the problem of early graft rejection, which could be corrected by a second transplant from the other parent, was observed. In the initial work of Reisner and colleagues[20] from 1983, all 3 patients who underwent TCD HSCT required repeat stem cell grafts as a result of early graft rejection. Several subsequent studies in which the rate of early graft rejection reached up to 30% and necessitated repeated transplantation confirmed these results.[2,38,41] This observation and the fear of increased mortality during the prolonged time of severe immune deficiency led to the use of somewhat reduced TCD, together with GVHD prophylaxis in the hope of achieving better graft engraftment.[23] The overall rate of 30% graft rejection is significantly higher than that observed when using a matched unrelated HSC donor.[41] In particular, NK+ SCID might lead to a higher rate of early graft rejection in the absence of conditioning treatment, unless prior maternal engraftment is present and the mother is the HSC donor.[7] However, although the main concern in early graft rejection is the prolonged period of vulnerability to infections, even with a higher incidence of graft rejection, requiring more than 1 transplant, overall survival was not inferior to that observed in other studies.[2]

T Cell Recovery

Twenty years ago T cell recovery was evaluated through the development of normal T cell counts and proliferative responses to phytohemagglutinin antigen, recall antigens such as purified protein derivative, and tetanus or allogeneic stimulators. In recent years attention has focused on long-lasting thymic activity that results in continuous production and development of a diverse T cell repertoire.

One method for evaluating T cell reconstitution and thymic function is the measurement of T cell receptor (TCR) rearrangement excisional circles (TRECs), which are found only in progenitor T cells undergoing TCR rearrangement and, for this reason, represent recently released naive T cells.[51]

In addition, based on differential T cell phenotypes, it has been shown that after HSCT, T cells may develop from 2 independent sources.[52,53] The first is mature memory donor T cells contained in the graft, expressing the surface marker CD45RO. These cells can undergo substantial and rapid expansion; mediate protective immunity early after transplantation but at the same time may induce GVHD. The second source is naive T cells, expressing the surface marker CD45RA, generated from thymic engrafted stem cells. The appearance of CD4+CD45RA+ T cells after transplantation represents thymic-derived naive T cells.

It is to be expected that a different pattern of T cell reconstitution will follow unmanipulated HSCT and TCD HSCT. The unmanipulated graft consists of progenitor cells and mature T cells. Therefore, T cell reconstitution is bimodal, with early expansion of mature T cells followed by a second wave of naive T cells resulting in neothymopoiesis. Although early T cell expansion supports rapid elevation of the lymphocyte count, it is unclear whether this T cell population provides sufficient immunity against infection, as these cells proliferate from a limited number of precursors and carry a TCR repertoire of limited diversity.[54]

Highly diverse naive T cells (CD45RA+) usually appear 3 to 6 months after transplantation and continue to increase during the first 2 years following transplantation. The initial time interval between transplantation and the appearance of naive T cells most likely reflects the time required for the complex process of intrathymic lymphoid maturation, and remains similarly independent of the donor type or stem cell manipulation.[55–58] One exception is unmanipulated, matched, unrelated donor graft, which in several studies in non-PID patients was thought to result in delayed immune reconstitution as a result of a higher incidence and severity of GVHD.[56,59]

Of several factors that were suspected of inhibiting T cell reconstitution, GVHD was found to be of great importance. It is thought that GVHD induces injury to host thymic and other lymphoid organs required for T cell reconstitution,[60] as reflected by the decreased TRECs number[56,59] and increased morbidity and mortality.[50,61] Prevention of GVHD in HSCT from other than an identical HSC donor is, therefore, of high priority and requires a more careful evaluation of the methods used for TCD.

Over the years, longer follow-up data have caused concern regarding the long-term results of T cell reconstitution following HSCT for PID. Patel and colleagues[57] and Sarzotti and colleagues[62] showed that despite satisfactory early T cell reconstitution, a rapid decline in thymic function follows HSCT in SCID patients. TRECs levels have declined to undetectable levels over a period of 14 years compared with approximately 80 years in a normal control patient, representing rapid thymic exhaustion. As most of the patients in these studies were transplanted with TCD haploidentical HSC donor, T cell depletion may be the cause of the apparent decline in thymopoiesis. However, other studies did not find similar results, and were able to demonstrate a positive correlation between continuous measurable TRECs level and the development of myeloid chimerism in the transplanted patient.[63,64] It has been suggested that early T cell reconstitution does not require marrow engraftment of donor CD34+ cells.[58] Therefore, it is possible that the lack of marrow engraftment is responsible for the late loss of thymic function in the absence of a continuous supply of marrow progenitor cells.[58,65] Although long-lasting thymic function was shown to correlate with myeloid donor chimerism,[60,61] which, in most cases, can be achieved only with myeloablative CR, patients in the studies describing thymic exhaustion did not receive any CR before transplantation.[57,59] The data may cause an uneasy dilemma for the patient and caregiver having to choose between an aggressive CR, which might result in reduced survival in the short-term, and long-term thymic exhaustion which might result in significant morbidity and mortality in the long-term. However, according to the available data (for some patients >18 years after TCD HSCT), the decline in thymic function was not associated with recurrent infection.[38,57,62]

B Cell Recovery

In general, B cell function in SCID patients does not develop as well as T cells following HSCT, and a substantial proportion of patients require immunoglobulin replacement therapy to prevent infections, even when using a related identical HSC graft in the absence of donor stem cell engraftment.[38,47]

Several factors have been shown to be associated with B cell recovery. T cell reconstitution 6 months after bone marrow transplant correlates with improved B cell function.[37] T−B−SCID was associated with a lower rate of B cell recovery, especially when no CR was given.[37,43] When evaluating B cell function in T−B+ SCID patients, engraftment of donor B cells offered the best chance for B cell recovery. However, chimerism was achieved only in a minority of the patients independent of HSC origin or nonmyeloablative CR.[66] Some SCID patients with normal B cells enjoy long-lasting functional host B cell function following the development of competent donor T cells.[47,66]

Of the different methods used for TCD, a comparison between CD34+ positive selection and anti-CD52 depletion showed an advantage for the anti-CD52–treated stem cells, as represented by a higher rate of normal IgG levels, a higher rate of class-switched memory B cells and a trend toward more complete B lymphocyte donor chimerism.[36] The findings could be explained by the hypothesis that positive stem cells selection (in contrast to T cell depletion) might result in removal of key stromal cells[67] or alloreactive NK cells from the graft and reduce engraftment.

Dependence on immunoglobulin replacement therapy tends to resolve in some patients over the years, independent of chimerism and SCID diagnosis.[50]

METHODS TO ENHANCE RECOVERY FOLLOWING TCD HSCT

The delayed T cell reconstitution following TCD HSCT is a major clinical problem as it is a period of profound immune deficiency during which the patient is exposed to lethal infectious complication. Several modalities have been suggested in an attempt to shorten the period of risk.

Haploidentical TCD HSCT in the neonatal period improved overall survival rate (95%) and might shorten the period between HSCT and normal T cell function.[42] Early CD34+ stem cell boost as a means to correct incomplete immune recovery was found to be beneficial when performed in the first year following transplantation.[68] Recently, several experimental methods using cell therapy have been suggested as a possible method of accelerating immune reconstitution, including treatment with nonalloreactive T cells, specific antiviral effector T cells and, hopefully in the future, ex vivo expanded T cell precursors to achieve rapid thymic seeding.[48,69]

One of the most encouraging results presented in recent years is the study of Dvorak and colleagues[70] describing a megadose CD34+ cell graft in a SCID patient. Administration of a megadose of CD34+ HSC has been reported to induce tolerance and enhance engraftment.[71] In accordance with this, a megadose of haploidentical CD34+ cells, together with a fixed number of CD3+ cells, without myeloablative chemotherapy, has been shown to result in a high rate of engraftment (73%), accelerated recovery of CD4 counts (1.2 months for CD4 >200) and a favorable overall survival rate of 87% despite relatively older age (median 5.7 months) and significant infections at the time of transplantation. However, there was a relatively high rate of grade II aGVHD (58%) and B cell function failed to develop in most patients.[70] Despite the small number of patients treated (15), the data are highly convincing and validate the haploidentical TCD HSC graft as the appropriate source for donor graft in the absence of an identical related donor.

SUMMARY

Several primary immune deficiency diseases can be cured by allogeneic HSCT. In the more severe form of otherwise lethal SCID disease, with the exception of experimental gene therapy, HSCT is the only curative treatment. It is well established that HSCT from an identical related donor offers the best survival outcome, lowest GVHD rate, and to some extent improved immune reconstitution. However, as a matched sibling donor is available for only a few patients, and because SCID is a medical emergency, a T cell depleted haploidentical stem cell donation from a close relative (mostly parents) has emerged as an alternative option.

Most of the data available for the assessment of TCD HSCT in PID patient is difficult to analyze as in many cases it involves multicenter studies, different cell preparations, and variable pre- and posttransplantation treatment. This is the result of several factors including the rarity of diseases, evolution of separation techniques, supportive treatments, CRs, progressive understanding of the different types of PIDs, and the clinical status of the patients which mandates a different approach from one patient to another. However, several issues are relevant when considering TCD HSCT.

With improved survival rates over the years,[38,40,70] TCD haploidentical HSCT is a reasonable alternative in the absence of an identical related donor. This is the case for SCID patients with T−B+ phenotype, but haploidentical TCD carries a much less favorable outcome when performed in T−B− SCID patients and in several other non-SCID PIDs compared with matched unrelated donor.[43,45]

GVHD and early immune reconstitution after TCD HSCT are 2 complicated issues that deserve specific consideration. Both have a significant effect on overall survival and, in a way, the 2 are directly linked to each other. GVHD is a significant risk factor for increased morbidity and mortality and impaired immune reconstitution.[40,47,50,56,60] Efforts have been made to reduce the incidence and severity of GVHD. However, posttransplant GVHD prophylaxis with immunosuppressive agents can be related to increased mortality and morbidity and perhaps delayed immune reconstitution. Given the low grade of GVHD following 3 log T cell depletion, it is difficult to justify the use of such treatments.[38] On the other hand, methods used to enhance engraftment and recovery, including myeloablative treatment and administration of grafts containing larger amounts of T cells, can aggravate GVHD, either through a direct effect of the transplanted T cells or, theoretically, through chemotherapy-mediated thymic injury and inferior tolerance induction. The authors, therefore, believe that the data support the compelling use of highly depleted stem cell grafts as a means of preventing GVHD, together with conservative patient support while waiting for immune reconstitution to develop. This suggestion is based, in part, on the observation that between 1980 and 1996 the North American groups, using largely an extensive T cell depletion with SBA and E-rosetting, attained better survival compared with that described by the European study, in which many patients received less rigorously deleted bone marrow and were therefore also treated by posttransplant GVHD prophylaxis. Furthermore, results in the European study following 1996, at which time T cell depletion was enhanced using positive selection of CD34 cells, reached the same survival rate as reported in the North American study.

Long-term immune reconstitution following TCD HSCT has remained a problem especially when considering humoral immunity. As B cell reconstitution was shown to be associated with B cell engraftment,[66] the use of myeloablative treatment to achieve the desirable donor chimerism could be considered. However, as such protocols were shown to be associated with increased early mortality and long-term clinical effects (especially in several types of SCID patients who are highly sensitive to irradiation and chemotherapy because of the basic genetic defect) and immunologic effects (possible thymic injury), it is difficult to justify such treatments over the more cautious approach avoiding the use of conditioning.

One approach to replace conventional conditioning could be the use of alloreactive NK cells, shown in mouse models to empty bone marrow niches[72] and thereby may enable engraftment of long-term HSCs, important for the establishment of long-lasting B and T cell reconstitution.

Over the years T cell depletion has become a synonym for haploidentical stem cell graft. However, because GVHD is an obvious problem when using an unmanipulated identical unrelated donor as a source for HSCT,[41] the use of T cell depleted stem cell graft should be considered, especially in situations in which haploidentical HSCT was shown to carry a less favorable outcome.

Finally, the encouraging results of a megadose of CD34+ haploidentical stem cell graft presented recently[60] makes this new approach highly compelling and attractive for use in other lethal PID conditions and with different stem cell donors. In particular, this approach could be used in conjunction with other tolerizing cells, such as anti–third-party CTLs[73,74] or immature dendritic cells,[75] in patients known to exhibit immune rejection.

Furthermore, early posttransplant T cell reconstitution might be enhanced by adoptive transfer of nonalloreactive T cells depleted of graft versus host reactivity ex vivo. In addition, recent results in leukemia patients suggest that combining effector donor T cells with donor natural T regulatory cells can effectively enhance immune reconstitution without GVHD (Martelli and colleagues, unpublished results, 2009).

TCD haploidentical HSCT has been shown to be a lifesaving procedure for SCID patients in the absence of an identical related donor. However, the multiplicity of reported studies and the diversity of PID diseases and methods used for treatment, stress the need for prospective studies in more homogeneous patient populations to evaluate the effect of the method used, the source of cells, and the extent of T cell depletion on the posttransplantation outcome.

REFERENCES

1. Geha RS, Notarangelo LD, Casanova JL, et al. The International Union of Immunological Societies (IUIS) primary immunodeficiency diseases (PID) classification committee. J Allergy Clin Immunol 2007;120(4):776.
2. Buckley RH. Molecular defects in human severe combined immunodeficiency and approaches to immune reconstitution. Annu Rev Immunol 2004;22:625–55.
3. Fischer A. Primary immunodeficiency diseases: an experimental model for molecular medicine. Lancet 2001;357(9271):1863–9.
4. Gatti R, Meuwissen H, Allen H, et al. Immunological reconstitution of sex-linked lymphopenic immunological deficiency. Lancet 1968;2(7583):1366.
5. Bortin M, Rimm A. Severe combined immunodeficiency disease. Characterization of the disease and results of transplantation. JAMA 1977;238(7):591–600.
6. Reisner Y, Kapoor N, Kirkpatrick D, et al. Transplantation for acute leukaemia with HLA-A and B nonidentical parental marrow cells fractionated with soybean agglutinin and sheep red blood cells. Lancet 1981;2(8242):327–31.

7. Griffith LM, Cowan MJ, Kohn DB, et al. Allogeneic hematopoietic cell transplantation for primary immune deficiency diseases: current status and critical needs. J Allergy Clin Immunol 2008;122(6):1087–96.
8. Zuckerman T, Rowe JM. Alternative donor transplantation in acute myeloid leukemia: which source and when? Curr Opin Hematol 2007;14:152–61.
9. Tiercy JM, Bujan-Lose M, Chapuis B, et al. Bone marrow transplantation with unrelated donors: what is the probability of identifying an HLA-A/B/Cw/DRB 1/B 3/B 5/DQB 1-matched donor? Bone Marrow Transplant (Basingstoke) 2000; 26(4):437–41.
10. Uphoff D. Preclusion of secondary phase of irradiation syndrome by inoculation of fetal hematopoietic tissue following lethal total-body x-irradiation. J Natl Cancer Inst 1958;20:625.
11. Yunis E, Good R, Smith J, et al. Protection of lethally irradiated mice by spleen cells from neonatally thymectomized mice. Proc Natl Acad Sci U S A 1974; 71(6):2544.
12. Bortin M, Saltzstein E. Graft-versus-host inhibition: fetal liver and thymus cells to minimize secondary disease. Transplantation 1969;8(5):712.
13. Korngold B, Sprent J. Lethal graft-versus-host disease after bone marrow transplantation across minor histocompatibility barriers in mice. Prevention by removing mature T cells from marrow. J Exp Med 1978;148(6):1687–98.
14. Reisner Y, Linker-Israeli M, Sharon N. Separation of mouse thymocytes into two subpopulations by the use of peanut agglutinin. Cell Immunol 1976;25(1):129–34.
15. Reisner Y, Ravid A, Sharon N. Use of soybean agglutinin for the separation of mouse B and T lymphocytes. Biochem Biophys Res Commun 1976;72(4):1585–91.
16. Reisner Y, Itzicovitch L, Meshorer A, et al. Hemopoietic stem cell transplantation using mouse bone marrow and spleen cells fractionated by lectins. Proc Natl Acad Sci U S A 1978;75(6):2933–6.
17. Reisner Y, Ikehara S, Hodes MZ, et al. Allogeneic hemopoietic stem cell transplantation using mouse spleen cells fractionated by lectins: in vitro study of cell fractions. Proc Natl Acad Sci U S A 1980;77(2):1164–8.
18. Reisner Y, Kapoor N, O'Reilly R, et al. Allogeneic bone marrow transplantation using stem cells fractionated by lectins: VI, in vitro analysis of human and monkey bone marrow cells fractionated by sheep red blood cells and soybean agglutinin. Lancet 1980;2(8208–8209):1320–4.
19. Reisner Y, Kapoor N, Good R, et al. Allogeneic bone marrow transplantation in mouse, monkey and man using lectin-separated grafts. In: Slavin S, editor. Tolerance in bone marrow and organ transplantation. Amsterdam (NY): Elsevier Science Publishing Co; 1984. p. 293.
20. Reisner Y, Kapoor N, Kirkpatrick D, et al. Transplantation for severe combined immunodeficiency with HLA-A, B, D, DR incompatible parental marrow cells fractionated by soybean agglutinin and sheep red blood cells. Blood 1983;61(2):341.
21. O'Reilly R, Kapoor N, Kirkpatrick D, et al. Transplantation for severe combined immunodeficiency using histoincompatible parental marrow fractionated by soybean agglutinin and sheep red blood cells: experience in six consecutive cases. Transplant Proc 1983;15(1):1431.
22. Friedrich W, Goldmann SF, Vetter U, et al. Immunoreconstitution in severe combined immunodeficiency after transplantation of HLA-identical, T-cell-depleted bone marrow. Lancet 1984;1(8380):761–4.
23. Fischer A, Durandy A, De Villartay J, et al. HLA-haploidentical bone marrow transplantation for severe combined immunodeficiency using E rosette fractionation and cyclosporine. Blood 1986;67(2):444.

24. Filipovich AH, McGlave PB, Ramsay NK, et al. Pretreatment of donor bone marrow with monoclonal antibody OKT3 for prevention of acute graft-versus-host disease in allogeneic histocompatible bone-marrow transplantation. Lancet 1982;1(8284):1266–9.
25. Hayward AR, Murphy S, Githens J, et al. Failure of a pan-reactive anti-T cell antibody, OKT 3, to prevent graft versus host disease in severe combined immunodeficiency. J Pediatr 1982;100(4):665–8.
26. Hale G, Bright S, Chumbley G, et al. Removal of T cells from bone marrow for transplantation: a monoclonal antilymphocyte antibody that fixes human complement. Blood 1983;62(4):873.
27. Frame JN, Collins NH, Cartagena T, et al. T cell depletion of human bone marrow. Comparison of Campath-1 plus complement, anti-T cell ricin A chain immunotoxin, and soybean agglutinin alone or in combination with sheep erythrocytes or immunomagnetic beads. Transplantation 1989;47(6):984–8.
28. Waldmann H, Hale G, Cividalli G, et al. Elimination of graft-versus-host disease by in-vitro depletion of alloreactive lymphocytes with a monoclonal rat anti-human lymphocyte antibody(CAMPATH-1). Lancet 1984;2(8401):483–5.
29. Apperley J, Jones L, Hale G, et al. Bone marrow transplantation for patients with chronic myeloid leukaemia: T-cell depletion with Campath-1 reduces the incidence of graft-versus-host disease but may increase the risk of leukaemic relapse. Bone Marrow Transplant 1986;1(1):53.
30. Hale G, Cobbold S, Waldmann H. T cell depletion with CAMPATH-1 in allogeneic bone marrow transplantation. Transplantation 1988;45(4):753.
31. Hale G, Zhang MJ, Bunjes D, et al. Improving the outcome of bone marrow transplantation by using CD52 monoclonal antibodies to prevent graft-versus-host disease and graft rejection. Blood 1998;92(12):4581.
32. Waldmann H, Hale G. CAMPATH: from concept to clinic. Philos Trans R Soc Lond B Biol Sci 2005;360(1461):1707.
33. Civin CI, Strauss LC, Fackler MJ, et al. Positive stem cell selection-basic science. Prog Clin Biol Res 1990;333:387–401 [discussion: 402].
34. Sutherland DR, Stewart AK, Keating A. CD34 antigen: molecular features and potential clinical applications. Stem Cells 1993;11(Suppl 3):50–7.
35. Shpall EJ, Gee A, Cagnoni PJ, et al. Stem cell isolation. Curr Opin Hematol 1995; 2(6):452–9.
36. Slatter MA, Brigham K, Dickinson AM, et al. Long-term immune reconstitution after anti-CD52-treated or anti-CD34-treated hematopoietic stem cell transplantation for severe T-lymphocyte immunodeficiency. J Allergy Clin Immunol 2008;121:361–7.
37. Haddad E, Landais P, Friedrich W, et al. Long-term immune reconstitution and outcome after HLA-nonidentical T-cell-depleted bone marrow transplantation for severe combined immunodeficiency: a European retrospective study of 116 patients. Blood 1998;91(10):3646.
38. Buckley RH, Schiff SE, Schiff RI, et al. Hematopoietic stem-cell transplantation for the treatment of severe combined immunodeficiency. N Engl J Med 1999;340(7): 508–16.
39. Small TN, Friedrich W, O'Reilly RJ. Hematopoietic cell transplantation for immunodeficiency diseases. In: Appelbaun FR, Forman SJ, Negrin S, et al, editors. Thomas' hematopoietic cell transplantation. 4th edition. Blackwell Publishing Ltd; 2009. p. 1105–24.
40. Antoine C, Müller S, Cant A, et al. Long-term survival and transplantation of haemopoietic stem cells for immunodeficiencies: report of the European experience 1968–99. Lancet 2003;361(9357):553–60.

41. Grunebaum E, Mazzolari E, Porta F, et al. Bone marrow transplantation for severe combined immune deficiency. JAMA 2006;295(5):508–18.

42. Myers LA, Patel DD, Puck JM, et al. Hematopoietic stem cell transplantation for severe combined immunodeficiency in the neonatal period leads to superior thymic output and improved survival. Blood 2002;99(3):872.

43. Bertrand Y, Landais P, Friedrich W, et al. Influence of severe combined immunodeficiency phenotype on the outcome of HLA non-identical, T-cell-depleted bone marrow transplantation: a retrospective European survey from the European Group for Bone Marrow Transplantation and the European Society for Immunodeficiency. J Pediatr 1999;134(6):740.

44. Booth C, Hershfield M, Notarangelo L, et al. Management options for adenosine deaminase deficiency. Proceedings of the EBMT satellite workshop (Hamburg, March 2006). Clin Immunol 2007;123(2):139–47.

45. Ozsahin H, Cavazzana-Calvo M, Notarangelo LD, et al. Long-term outcome following hematopoietic stem-cell transplantation in Wiskott-Aldrich syndrome: collaborative study of the European Society for Immunodeficiencies and European Group for Blood and Marrow Transplantation. Blood 2008;111(1): 439.

46. Filipovich AH, Stone JV, Tomany SC, et al. Impact of donor type on outcome of bone marrow transplantation for Wiskott-Aldrich syndrome: collaborative study of the International Bone Marrow Transplant Registry and the National Marrow Donor Program. Blood 2001;97(6):1598.

47. Cowan MJ, Neven B, Cavazanna-Calvo M, et al. Hematopoietic stem cell transplantation for severe combined immunodeficiency diseases. Biol Blood Marrow Transplant 2008;14(1S):73–80.

48. Cavazzana-Calvo M, André-Schmutz I, Dal Cortivo L, et al. Immune reconstitution after haematopoietic stem cell transplantation: obstacles and anticipated progress. Curr Opin Immunol 2009;21:544–8.

49. Scaradavou A, Carrier C, Mollen N, et al. Detection of maternal DNA in placental/umbilical cord blood by locus-specific amplification of the noninherited maternal HLA gene. Blood 1996;88(4):1494.

50. Neven B, Leroy S, Decaluwe H, et al. Long-term outcome after hematopoietic stem cell transplantation of a single-center cohort of 90 patients with severe combined immunodeficiency. Blood 2009;113(17):4114.

51. Douek DC, McFarland RD, Keiser PH, et al. Changes in thymic function with age and during the treatment of HIV infection. Nature 1998;396(6712):690–5.

52. Mackall C, Granger L, Sheard M, et al. T-cell regeneration after bone marrow transplantation: differential CD45 isoform expression on thymic-derived versus thymic-independent progeny. Blood 1993;82(8):2585.

53. Dumont-Girard F, Roux E, van Lier RA, et al. Reconstitution of the T-cell compartment after bone marrow transplantation: restoration of the repertoire by thymic emigrants. Blood 1998;92(11):4464.

54. Roux E, Helg C, Dumont-Girard F, et al. Analysis of T-cell repopulation after allogeneic bone marrow transplantation: significant differences between recipients of T-cell depleted and unmanipulated grafts. Blood 1996;87(9):3984.

55. Small T, Papadopoulos E, Boulad F, et al. Comparison of immune reconstitution after unrelated and related T-cell-depleted bone marrow transplantation: effect of patient age and donor leukocyte infusions. Blood 1999;93(2):467.

56. Weinberg K, Blazar BR, Wagner JE, et al. Factors affecting thymic function after allogeneic hematopoietic stem cell transplantation. Blood 2001;97(5): 1458.

57. Patel DD, Gooding ME, Parrott RE, et al. Thymic function after hematopoietic stem-cell transplantation for the treatment of severe combined immunodeficiency. N Engl J Med 2000;342(18):1325–32.
58. Muller SM, Kohn T, Schulz AS, et al. Similar pattern of thymic-dependent T-cell reconstitution in infants with severe combined immunodeficiency after human leukocyte antigen (HLA)-identical and HLA-nonidentical stem cell transplantation. Blood 2000;96(13):4344.
59. Lewin SR, Heller G, Zhang L, et al. Direct evidence for new T-cell generation by patients after either T-cell-depleted or unmodified allogeneic hematopoietic stem cell transplantations. Blood 2002;100(6):2235.
60. Dulude G, Roy DC, Perreault C. The effect of graft-versus-host disease on T cell production and homeostasis. J Exp Med 1999;189(8):1329–42.
61. Hazenberg MD, Otto SA, de Pauw ES, et al. T-cell receptor excision circle and T-cell dynamics after allogeneic stem cell transplantation are related to clinical events. Blood 2002;99(9):3449.
62. Sarzotti M, Patel DD, Li X, et al. T cell repertoire development in humans with SCID after nonablative allogeneic marrow transplantation 1. J Immunol 2003; 170(5):2711–8.
63. Borghans JA, Bredius RG, Hazenberg MD, et al. Early determinants of long-term T-cell reconstitution after hematopoietic stem cell transplantation for severe combined immunodeficiency. Blood 2006;108(2):763.
64. Cavazzana-Calvo M, Carlier F, Le Deist F, et al. Long-term T-cell reconstitution after hematopoietic stem-cell transplantation in primary T-cell-immunodeficient patients is associated with myeloid chimerism and possibly the primary disease phenotype. Blood 2007;109(10):4575.
65. Frey J, Ernst B, Surh C, et al. Thymus-grafted SCID mice show transient thymopoiesis and limited depletion of V beta 11 T cells. J Exp Med 1992;175(4): 1067–71.
66. Haddad E, Deist FL, Aucouturier P, et al. Long-term chimerism and B-cell function after bone marrow transplantation in patients with severe combined immunodeficiency with B cells: a single-center study of 22 patients. Blood 1999;94(8):2923.
67. Slatter M, Bhattacharya A, Flood T, et al. Polysaccharide antibody responses are impaired post bone marrow transplantation for severe combined immunodeficiency, but not other primary immunodeficiencies. Bone Marrow Transplant 2003;32(2):225–9.
68. Booth C, Ribeil JA, Audat F, et al. CD34 stem cell top-ups without conditioning after initial haematopoietic stem cell transplantation for correction of incomplete haematopoietic and immunological recovery in severe congenital immunodeficiencies. Br J Haematol 2006;135(4):533–7.
69. André-Schmutz I, Six E, Bonhomme D, et al. Shortening the immunodeficient period after hematopoietic stem cell transplantation. Immunol Res 2009;44(1): 54–60.
70. Dvorak CC, Hung GY, Horn B, et al. Megadose CD34 cell grafts improve recovery of T cell engraftment but not B cell immunity in patients with severe combined immunodeficiency disease undergoing haplocompatible nonmyeloablative transplantation. Biol Blood Marrow Transplant 2008;14(10):1125–33.
71. Rachamim N, Gan J, Segall H, et al. Tolerance induction by "megadose" hematopoietic transplants: donor-type human CD34 stem cells induce potent specific reduction of host anti-donor cytotoxic T lymphocyte precursors in mixed lymphocyte culture. Transplantation 1998;65(10):1386–93.

72. Ruggeri L, Capanni M, Urbani E, et al. Effectiveness of donor natural killer cell alloreactivity in mismatched hematopoietic transplants. Science 2002; 295(5562):2097.
73. Bachar-Lustig E, Reich-Zeliger S, Reisner Y. Anti-third-party veto CTLs overcome rejection of hematopoietic allografts: synergism with rapamycin and BM cell dose. Blood 2003;102(6):1943.
74. Edelshtein Y, Ophir E, Bachar-Lustig E, et al. Ex-vivo acquisition of central memory phenotype is critical for tolerance induction by donor anti-3rd party CD8 T cells in allogeneic bone marrow transplantation. Blood (ASH Annual Meeting Abstracts) 2008;112:2323.
75. Yu P, Xiong S, He Q, et al. Induction of allogeneic mixed chimerism by immature dendritic cells and bone marrow transplantation leads to prolonged tolerance to major histocompatibility complex disparate allografts. Immunology 2009;127(4): 500–11.

Bone Marrow Transplantation Using HLA-Matched Unrelated Donors for Patients Suffering from Severe Combined Immunodeficiency

Eyal Grunebaum, MD, Chaim M. Roifman, MD, FRCPC, FCACB*

KEYWORDS

- Immunodeficiency • Transplantation
- Unrelated • Long-term

Severe combined immunodeficiency (SCID) is a heterogeneous group of inherited diseases characterized by significantly impaired T-cell immunity that leads to death in infancy. The diagnosis of SCID relies on distinct clinical manifestations and laboratory features, and ideally is confirmed by the identification of mutations in genes known to be critical for T lineage development and function. Complete cure can be attained in the majority of patients suffering from SCID by using allogeneic bone marrow transplantation (BMT). The best outcome is achieved by family-related genotypically HLA-identical donors (RID). Among populations with high consanguinity marriage, RID account for the majority of transplants for SCID[1]; however, in most European and North American populations, RID are found for only 15% to 25% of the patients.[2,3] BMT using phenotypically HLA-matched family-related donors (PMD) have resulted in a relatively high success rate[4]; however, PMD are not frequently found.[2] The lack of RID or PMD for more than 75% of SCID patients led many groups to search for alternative sources, such as parents who are often HLA-haploidentical donors (HID) or HLA-matched unrelated donors (MUD).

The first attempt to treat SCID with unmodified MUD transplant was performed in 1973. A patient diagnosed with SCID, whose similarly affected sister died previously

Division of Immunology and Allergy, Department of Pediatrics, The Hospital for Sick Children, 555 University Avenue, Toronto, Ontario M5G 1X8, Canada
* Corresponding author.
E-mail address: chaim.roifman@sickkids.ca (C.M. Roifman).

Immunol Allergy Clin N Am 30 (2010) 63–73
doi:10.1016/j.iac.2009.11.001
0889-8561/10/$ – see front matter © 2010 Published by Elsevier Inc.

immunology.theclinics.com

after receiving a transplant from her HLA-haploidentical parent, underwent BMT from a partially MUD found among 800 normal individuals registered in Denmark. The patient achieved durable engraftment with complete hematopoietic and immunologic reconstitution, but suffered from skin and oral mucosa chronic graft versus host disease (GvHD).[5]

Difficulties finding HLA-matched unrelated donors and the lack of adequate means to control GvHD, together with the increased availability of T-cell depleted HID BMT in the early 1980s resulted in limited use of MUD BMT for SCID. However, it soon became apparent that with some exceptions,[6] the success rate of HID BMT consistently hovered around 50% at best, regardless of the T-cell depletion method[1,2,7–13] (D. Kohn, Los Angeles, California, personal communication, 2006; L. Notarangelo, Brescia, Italy, personal communication, 2006).

During the late 1980s, several events including the disappointment from HID BMT for SCID, the surge in the number of bone marrow donor registries (**Fig. 1**), and the development of efficient medications to control GvHD, such as cyclosporine A (CsA), prompted Dr Roifman to systematically explore the systematic use of MUD BMT for SCID in their center. Therefore, in 1987, Dr Roifman created a protocol for MUD BMT in SCID. The protocol included strict patient isolation in private HEPA-filtered rooms from diagnosis until discharge, intensive pretransplant antimicrobial management with intravenous immunoglobulins (to maintain IgG ≥6 g/L), *Pneumocystis jiroveci* pneumonia prophylaxis, close Herpes virus group surveillance, and nutritional support. Pretransplant conditioning consisted of oral or intravenous busulfan in 16 doses over 4 days (total amount ranging from 16 to 20 mg/kg), in accordance with busulfan blood levels, followed by a 4-day course of cyclophosphamide. Patients received 3 to 5 × 10^8 nucleated cells per kilogram body weight from bone marrow that was unmodified except for volume reduction and plasma removal in blood group mismatch. The amount of nucleated bone marrow harvested from the adult donors was often greater than that required for the infant SCID, therefore excess bone marrow was frozen as backup for graft failure. Patients also received aggressive GvHD prophylaxis and treatment, detailed later in this article, as well as granulocyte-macrophage colony stimulating factor or granulocyte colony stimulating factor from the day of transplant (or day +5 in some cases). This protocol led to improved engraftment and patient survival, which was summarized in 2000 by Dalal and colleagues.[14]

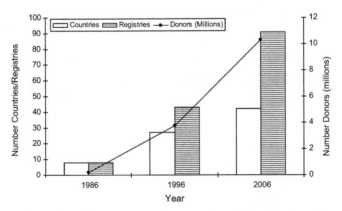

Fig. 1. Increase in registered bone marrow donors and registries. Number of countries that have bone marrow registries, number of registries, and number of donors (in millions) registered in 1986, 1996, and 2006.

Among the first 15 patients with SCID and CID in the authors' center who underwent BMT from HLA-matched or 1 non-DR antigen mismatched unrelated donors, survival was 73.3% with a mean follow-up of 47.4 months (range 18–101 months). All patients had leukocytes engraftment, which were demonstrated to be 100% donor by restriction length fragment polymorphism. Deaths were directly attributed to GvHD disease in 2 patients, while the third patient died of *Streptococcus viridans* sepsis and bone marrow aplasia 1 year after transplant, presumably also due to GvHD.

Other centers using MUD BMT for SCID also achieved excellent engraftment, with survival ranging from 71.5% to 83.3%.[13,15,16] These reports suffered from drawbacks such as the small number of patients in each study, which represented only single centers and lacked long-term evaluation of immune reconstitution. Therefore, in 2004 the authors initiated a study comparing the outcome of 94 patients with SCID who received BMT from 1990 until 2004 at the Hospital for Sick Children, Toronto, Canada and Brescia, Italy. Of importance, this study contained the largest group of patients with SCID to have undergone MUD BMT. The study also provided a unique opportunity for direct and detailed comparison of 40 patients transplanted using HLA-mismatched related donors (MMRD), mostly HID, with 41 patients transplanted with MUD.[3] The clinical presentation, age of diagnosis, molecular diagnosis, and gender, as well as maintenance prior to and after BMT were similar in both centers and among both transplant groups (**Table 1**). Of note is that among 9 patients initially considered as clinically unstable, 4 could be stabilized and only a few required "rush" BMT. The latter emphasizes that while the diagnosis and initial treatment of SCID is a medical emergency, once patients have been stabilized, the BMT itself should be performed with the best available donor.

The median time from diagnosis to MUD BMT in the authors' study was only 4 months, which is shorter than previously reported, probably because of the expansion and improvement of bone marrow registries. Still, the median time from diagnosis to MMRD BMT was only 2 months. However, 30% of the MMRD recipients lost the graft and required repeat BMT (see later discussion), therefore the actual median time from

Table 1
Comparison between pretransplant features of SCID patients who received MMRD or MUD BMT

	MUD (N = 41)	MMRD (N = 40)	P
Males/females	28/13	29/11	0.78
Diagnosis before 3 mo of age	11	14	0.43
Diagnosis between 3 and 12 mo of age	27	25	0.75
Diagnosis after 12 mo of age	3	1	0.32
Failure to thrive	13	8	0.17
Lung disease	14	19	0.16
Diarrhea	5	9	0.17
Rash	6	8	0.36
Candida	6	7	0.48
Unstable clinical condition	4	5	0.48
No clinical abnormalities	8	6	0.40
T−B+NK− immune phenotype	14	16	0.29
T−B−NK+ immune phenotype	12	15	0.20

diagnosis to the final MMRD BMT increased to 3 months, eliminating some of the potential disadvantage of MUD.

Most importantly, long-term survival was significantly better after MUD BMT than after MMRD BMT (80.5% compared with 52.5%, respectively), as demonstrated in **Fig. 2**. The survival after MUD BMT was similar in Toronto and Brescia, suggesting that the outcome was not specific to one center. In addition, there was no difference in outcome whether BMT was performed between 1990 and 1997 or between 1998 and 2004, suggesting lack of effect by change of antimicrobial or supportive management over the years. Survival of patients with B– SCID phenotype, associated previously with poor prognosis,[17] was not different to that in B+ SCID, nor did the specific molecular defect causing SCID affect survival. Moreover, as described later by the authors[18] and by others,[19] patients with Omenn syndrome or residual T cells (T+) SCID also had excellent outcome after MUD BMT, which is discussed in an article elsewhere in this issue.

Engraftment of hematopoietic cell lineages was robust after MUD BMT (**Fig. 3**), with all patients demonstrating 100% donor leukocyte engraftment by 1 month after transplant. Graft failure was observed in only 3 of the 41 (7.3%) patients who received MUD BMT. The authors repeated BMT in 2 of these patients using frozen bone marrow from the unrelated donors following conditioning with cyclophosphamide and total lymphoid irradiation. Both patients achieved complete donor engraftment, which persists 10 and 8 years after transplant, respectively. In marked contrast, a significantly ($P = .009$) higher frequency of donor graft failure was observed after MMRD BMT (**Fig. 4**), with 12 patients (30%) requiring a second transplant. Repeated MMRD BMT led to donor engraftment in only 4 patients. Two patients underwent a third MMRD BMT, one of which was successful. Increased frequency of graft failures after MMRD BMT in patients with SCID were also reported by other centers. Three of 16 patients in Florida also required repeat transplant, with only 1 of them surviving,[11] while 8 of 24 patients in San Francisco required more than 1 MMRD transplant.[7] Graft failure was particularly common when myeloablative conditioning was withheld or significantly altered, although some patients in the authors' study, as well as in other reports, failed to engraft after MMRD despite myeloablation, possibly because the T-cell depletion and ex vivo manipulation can also affect hematopoietic progenitors.

The ultimate purpose of BMT for SCID is to fully restore immune function and return patients to normal unrestricted lives indefinitely. Therefore, the authors were particularly interested in long-term immune reconstitution, 2 or more years after BMT, when

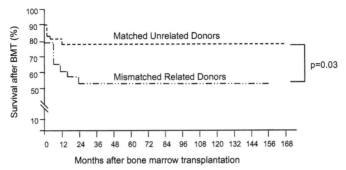

Fig. 2. Survival of patients with SCID who received BMT from MUD or MMRD. Percentage of patients surviving after MUD or MMRD BMT. For patients who received multiple transplants, survival was calculated from the date of the last transplant.

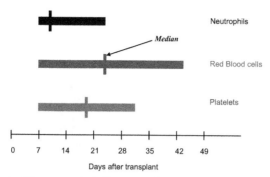

Fig. 3. Engraftment of hematopoietic lineages after MUD BMT for SCID. The numbers of days required to achieve engraftment of neutrophils (absolute neutrophil count >500/μL), red blood cells (last red blood cells transfusion), and platelets (platelets >20,000/μL) after MUD BMT for patients with SCID at the Hospital for Sick Children, Toronto, Canada.

most patients had stopped immune suppressive medications. Again, better results were achieved with MUD BMT compared with MMRD BMT, with complete donor lymphocyte engraftment in 88.5% and 66%, respectively. Lymphocyte subsets, in vitro responses of T lymphocytes to mitogens and T-cell receptor excision circles, which represent new thymic emigrants, were normal in all but one of the patients tested after MUD BMT. Similar results were also found after MMRD BMT. In contrast, normal distribution of T-cell receptor variable beta-chain expression was demonstrated in 18 (94.7%) of 19 MUD BMT patients, compared with only 11 (61.1%) of 18 MMRD BMT patients (**Fig. 5**). The latter findings are in agreement with other reports detailing immune dysfunction following MMRD for SCID. Among 11 patients in the Netherlands that received HID BMT for SCID, 4 were considered to have poor long-term T-cell immune reconstitution.[20] The abnormal T-cell immune reconstitution might be related to the rigorous depletion of donor T cells required for HID BMT. Of importance, the authors continue to monitor the patients every year, and have observed normal immune function in all patients even 20 years after MUD BMT (**Table 2**).

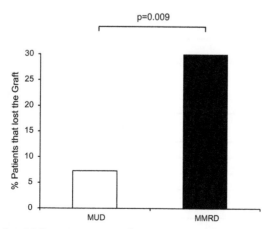

Fig. 4. Graft loss after MUD or MMRD BMT for SCID. Percentage of patients with SCID that lost donor lymphocyte engraftment after MUD or MMRD BMT.

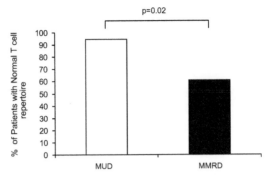

Fig. 5. T-cell receptor repertoire after MUD or MMRD BMT for SCID. Percentage of patients with SCID that achieved normal T-cell repertoire, as determined by T-cell receptor variable beta chain expression, after MUD or MMRD BMT.

Patients with SCID are particularly prone to respiratory track infections. Indeed, lower respiratory tract infections and pneumonitis, most frequently caused by viral or fungal infections, occurred in 14 SCID patients after MMRD BMT and was the cause of death in 12 patients (**Fig. 6**). In contrast, only 3 SCID patients who received MUD BMT experienced pneumonitis, which was the cause of death in only one patient. Other infections were also infrequent among MUD BMT recipients, possibly because of the rapid and robust immune reconstitution described earlier. Of note, veno-occlusive disease of the liver, which has been reported in some patients with SCID undergoing BMT,[13,21] was not detected in any of the authors' patients despite their use of myeloablative conditioning, possibly because myeloablation is administered when the patients were clinically stable. Mucositis and hemorrhagic cystitis, commonly seen with the use of busulfan and cyclophosphamide, similarly have been rare and relatively mild among SCID patients undergoing MUD BMT.

The use of MUD was expected to be associated with significant GvHD; Therefore, all the authors' patients received GvHD prophylaxis, which consisted of intravenous CsA and methylprednisolone (MPO). CsA (3 mg/kg/d) was initially given from the day before transplant although currently the authors begin CsA as early as 3 days before transplant. CsA doses were adjusted to maintain a trough level of 150 to 200 µg/L. MPO (2 mg/kg/d) was given from the day of the transplant divided into 2 doses. The

Table 2
Long-term immune reconstitution after MUD BMT at the Hospital for Sick Children, Toronto, Canada

	No. of Patients Tested	Percent of Patients with Normal Results
Complete donor lymph engraftment	32	100%
T-cell numbers	22	100%
T-cell mitogenic responses	20	100%
Antibody production	21	100%
T-cell receptor excision circles	15	100%
T-cell receptor V-beta diversity	13	100%

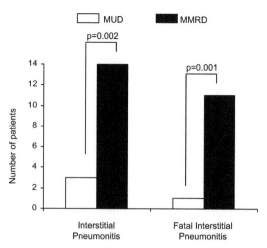

Fig. 6. Pneumonitis after MUD or MMRD BMT for SCID. Number of patients with SCID that suffered interstitial pneumonitis and died of interstitial pneumonitis after MUD or MMRD BMT.

authors tried adding methotrexate, 10 mg/m^2 on days 3, 6, 11, and 18 in a few SCID patients, as suggested by other investigators[22]; however, the lack of clear benefit and the frequent need to omit several doses of methotrexate because of liver abnormalities led to the removal of methotrexate from the protocol. Despite the aggressive GvHD prophylaxis, acute GvHD did develop in 73.1% of the 41 SCID patients who received MUD BMT in Toronto and Brescia. Although acute GvHD was transient and limited to the skin in most SCID patients after MUD BMT, it was the major cause of death in these patients. Therefore, the authors were particularly aggressive in treating acute GvHD and have treated patients who developed grade II or higher acute GvHD with high-dose steroid pulses. Among the 16 SCID patients in the authors' center that developed acute GvHD after MUD BMT, 13 had grade II or higher acute GvHD.[23] These patients were treated with high-dose MPO for 3 days, each followed by gradual dose reduction. Ten of these 13 patients received a pulse of 30 mg/kg/d, whereas 3 patients were given lower doses (10–20 mg/kg/d). Of note, 2 of the 3 patients who received the lower doses of MPO pulse as well as 2 of the patients who had low-grade GvHD and were not pulsed developed chronic GvHD, whereas none of the patients who received high-dose MPO pulse therapy developed chronic GvHD ($P = .015$). Pulse therapy was given to patients at a mean of 13.5 days after BMT (range, 7–35 days) and a mean of 0.6 days after the first symptoms of acute GvHD were apparent (range, 0–7 days). This treatment was effective in reversing 12 of 14 episodes of grade II or higher acute GvHD (one patient received 2 steroid pulses). Episodes of acute GvHD involving multiple organs including skin, liver, and gut were less likely to fully respond to MPO pulse therapy. The 2 patients who failed to respond to pulse therapy also failed other acute GvHD medications and eventually succumbed to GvHD. Patients usually tolerated the MPO pulse regimen without significant adverse effects. An increase in blood pressure (as determined by the need to add antihypertension medications to keep systolic blood pressure ≤95th percentile) was the most common side effect. The increased blood pressure may have also contributed to the development of hypertrophic cardiomyopathy, which reversed after discontinuation of MPO.[24] Most patients, however, already had hypertension before the pulse therapy due to the use of standard dose steroids and CsA. Other adverse effects included hyperglycemia, which was evident in 12.5% of patients. Four patients who received MPO had gastrointestinal bleeding, which was likely related to acute gut GvHD. Of importance, 2 SCID patients who received anti T-cell specific antibodies for acute GvHD developed Epstein-Barr virus–associated posttransplant lymphoproliferative disease and lymphoma, which was fatal in one patient, emphasizing again that high-dose steroids may be the best treatment for SCID patients failing GvHD prophylaxis.

The authors' aggressive treatment of acute GvHD may have also been the reason for the good outcome, that is, although the frequency of acute GvHD after MUD BMT was significantly higher than after MMRD BMT (P = .009), the frequency of grade III and IV GvHD after MUD BMT was not different than after MMRD BMT (**Fig. 7**). GvHD after the first few months of transplant, which often involved the skin and mucous membranes, was diagnosed in 8 of 35 patients after MUD BMT, a frequency that was not significantly different to that found among MMRD BMT recipients (P = .06). After MUD BMT, one patient developed fatal GvHD of the liver, and another had bone marrow failure that may have been associated with chronic GvHD. Chronic GvHD was the cause of death in one child after MMRD BMT. GvHD tended to surface when immune suppressive medications were changed from intravenous to oral or when prednisone doses were tapered rapidly (>5 mg/wk), particularly if they were not monitored closely by physicians experienced with such patients; the authors therefore tend to reduce immune suppression very gradually (not more than 25% of the total dose on alternate days) over extended periods (not more frequent than once every 2 weeks), which often continues for 6 to 12 months.

Other immune-mediated disorders that occurred during the 2 years after MUD BMT included autoimmune hematopoietic cytopenia (6 patients) and myocarditis (2 patients), while polymyositis and bronchiolitis obliterans were each diagnosed in one patient. Hematopoietic cytopenia was documented in 5 SCID patients after MMRD BMT. In contrast to the high frequency of complications shortly after transplant, late complications after MUD BMT were rare. Three patients had chronic GvHD that persisted for up to 7 years after MUD BMT, which resolved in 2. One of these patients died 6 years after transplant from an unknown cause. Significant neurologic defects after MUD BMT were found in 2 SCID patients, one who already suffered from neurologic abnormalities before transplant and the other who had a defect in the DNA Ligase IV gene, which is known to cause such abnormalities.[25]

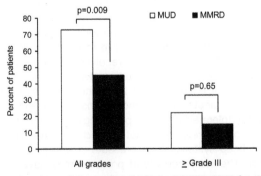

Fig. 7. Acute graft versus host disease after MUD or MMRD BMT for SCID. Percentage of patients with SCID that suffered acute graft versus host disease or grade III and higher acute graft versus host disease after MUD or MMRD BMT.

The low frequency of late complications that the authors observed after MUD BMT is in stark contrast to a recent report.[26] Among 90 patients who were 2 or more years after BMT (57% after MMRD, 24.5% after RID, 16.5% after PMD, and 2% after MUD), 10 patients had persistent chronic GvHD and 12 patients displayed other immune-mediated complications. Three patients died of chronic GvHD and related infectious complications, while 5 died of other immune-mediated disorders. A detailed description of 20 long-term survivors after MMRD BMT in Brescia[10] similarly revealed immune-mediated complications in 5 patients (25%). There were also 5 patients (25%) who suffered from neurologic abnormalities.[10] In contrast, among the 10 long-term survivors after MUD BMT in Brescia, only one patient had immune-mediated complications and none had neurologic abnormalities.

The data described clearly show that MUD BMT is an excellent alternative source of hematopoietic stem cells for patients with SCID. Therefore, in the authors' center, for SCID patients who do not have an RID or PMD and are clinically stable or can be stabilized through intensive care, a search for a MUD is initiated. For the few patients who cannot be stabilized, the option of HID would be offered. For patients for whom the authors failed to find a MUD, particularly if they are from populations not well represented in donor registries, HID does remain an option, although it is expected that the percentage of such patients will decrease with the expansion of bone marrow registries and cord blood banks. In addition, advances in HLA analysis and better management of GvHD are expected to further improve outcome of MUD BMT for SCID.

In conclusion, the close to 80% long-term survival, excellent immune reconstitution, and normal quality of life that the authors' and other groups have demonstrated after MUD BMT suggest that in the absence of RID or PMD, MUD BMT should be offered to patients suffering from SCID.

ACKNOWLEDGMENTS

The Audrey and Donald Campbell, The Jeffery Modell Foundation, and The Canadian Immunodeficiency Society for their support of Dr Roifman and data collection at the Hospital for Sick Children, Toronto, Canada. Brenda Reid, Advanced Practice Nurse in the division of Immunology, Hospital for Sick Children, Toronto, Canada. The dedicated team of physicians, nurses, pharmacists, dieticians and social workers at the Blood and Marrow Transplant Unit, and the post-BMT outpatient clinic for SCID, Hospital for Sick Children, Toronto, Canada.

REFERENCES

1. Al-Ghonaium A. Stem cell transplantation for primary immunodeficiencies: King Faisal Specialist Hospital experience from 1993 to 2006. Bone Marrow Transplant 2008;42(Suppl 1):S53–6.
2. Antoine C, Müller S, Cant A, et al. European Group for Blood and Marrow Transplantation; European Society for Immunodeficiency. Long-term survival and transplantation of haemopoietic stem cells for immunodeficiencies: report of the European experience 1968–99. Lancet 2003;361(9357):553–60.
3. Grunebaum E, Mazzolari E, Porta F, et al. Bone marrow transplantation for severe combined immune deficiency. JAMA 2006;295(5):508–18.
4. Caillat-Zucman S, Le Deist F, Haddad E, et al. Impact of HLA matching on outcome of hematopoietic stem cell transplantation in children with inherited diseases: a single-center comparative analysis of genoidentical, haploidentical or unrelated donors. Bone Marrow Transplant 2004;33(11):1089–95.

5. O'Reilly RJ, Dupont B, Pahwa S, et al. Reconstitution in severe combined immunodeficiency by transplantation of marrow from an unrelated donor. N Engl J Med 1977;297(24):1311–8.

6. Buckley RH, Schiff SE, Schiff RI, et al. Hematopoietic stem-cell transplantation for the treatment of severe combined immunodeficiency. N Engl J Med 1999;340(7):508–16.

7. Dror Y, Gallagher R, Wara DW, et al. Immune reconstitution in severe combined immunodeficiency disease after lectin-treated, T-cell-depleted haplocompatible bone marrow transplantation. Blood 1993;81(8):2021–30.

8. Fischer A, Landais P, Friedrich W, et al. European experience of bone-marrow transplantation for severe combined immunodeficiency. Lancet 1990;336(8719): 850–4.

9. Gennery AR, Dickinson AM, Brigham K, et al. CAMPATH-1M T-cell depleted BMT for SCID: long-term follow-up of 19 children treated 1987-98 in a single center. Cytotherapy 2001;3(3):221–32.

10. Mazzolari E, Forino C, Guerci S, et al. Long-term immune reconstitution and clinical outcome after stem cell transplantation for severe T-cell immunodeficiency. J Allergy Clin Immunol 2007;120(4):892–9.

11. Petrovic A, Dorsey M, Miotke J, et al. Hematopoietic stem cell transplantation for pediatric patients with primary immunodeficiency diseases at All Children's Hospital/University of South Florida. Immunol Res 2009;44(1–3):169–78.

12. Roifman CM, Grunebaum E, Dalal I, et al. Matched unrelated bone marrow transplant for severe combined immunodeficiency. Immunol Res 2007;38(1–3): 191–200.

13. Tsuji Y, Imai K, Kajiwara M, et al. Hematopoietic stem cell transplantation for 30 patients with primary immunodeficiency diseases: 20 years experience of a single team. Bone Marrow Transplant 2006;37(5):469–77.

14. Dalal I, Reid B, Doyle J, et al. Matched unrelated bone marrow transplantation for combined immunodeficiency. Bone Marrow Transplant 2000;25(6):613–21.

15. Filipovich AH, Shapiro RS, Ramsay NK, et al. Unrelated donor bone marrow transplantation for correction of lethal congenital immunodeficiencies. Blood 1992;80(1):270–6.

16. Rao K, Amrolia PJ, Jones A, et al. Improved survival after unrelated donor bone marrow transplantation in children with primary immunodeficiency using a reduced-intensity conditioning regimen. Blood 2005;105(2):879–85.

17. Bertrand Y, Landais P, Friedrich W, et al. Influence of severe combined immunodeficiency phenotype on the outcome of HLA non-identical, T-cell-depleted bone marrow transplantation: a retrospective European survey from the European group for bone marrow transplantation and the European society for immunodeficiency. J Pediatr 1999;134(6):740–8.

18. Roifman CM, Somech R, Grunebaum E. Matched unrelated bone marrow transplant for T+ combined immunodeficiency. Bone Marrow Transplant 2008;41(11): 947–52.

19. Mazzolari E, Moshous D, Forino C, et al. Hematopoietic stem cell transplantation in Omenn syndrome: a single-center experience. Bone Marrow Transplant 2005; 36(2):107–14.

20. Borghans JA, Bredius RG, Hazenberg MD, et al. Early determinants of long-term T-cell reconstitution after hematopoietic stem cell transplantation for severe combined immunodeficiency. Blood 2006;108(2):763–9.

21. Bhattacharya A, Slatter MA, Chapman CE, et al. Single centre experience of umbilical cord stem cell transplantation for primary immunodeficiency. Bone Marrow Transplant 2005;36(4):295–9.

22. Storb R, Deeg HJ, Whitehead J, et al. Methotrexate and cyclosporine compared with cyclosporine alone for prophylaxis of acute graft versus host disease after marrow transplantation for leukemia. N Engl J Med 1986;314(12):729–35.
23. Somech R, Kavadas FD, Atkinson A, et al. High-dose methylprednisolone is effective in the management of acute graft-versus-host disease in severe combined immune deficiency. J Allergy Clin Immunol 2008;122(6):1215–6.
24. Bulley SR, Benson L, Grunebaum E, et al. Cardiac chamber hypertrophy following hematopoietic stem cell transplantation for primary immunodeficiency. Biol Blood Marrow Transplant 2008;14(2):229–35.
25. Grunebaum E, Bates A, Roifman CM. Omenn syndrome is associated with mutations in DNA ligase IV. J Allergy Clin Immunol 2008;122(6):1219–20.
26. Neven B, Leroy S, Decaluwe H, et al. Long-term outcome after hematopoietic stem cell transplantation of a single-center cohort of 90 patients with severe combined immunodeficiency. Blood 2009;113(17):4114–24.

Pathogenesis and Management of Graft-versus-Host Disease

Sung W. Choi, MD[a],*, John E. Levine, MD[b],
James L.M. Ferrara, MD, DSc[c]

KEYWORDS

- Acute graft-versus-host disease
- Chronic graft-versus-host disease
- Hematopoietic cell transplantation • GVHD

Allogeneic hematopoietic cell transplantation (HCT) is an important therapeutic option for various malignant and nonmalignant conditions.[1] The indication for its use has expanded, especially among older patients, in recent years through novel strategies using donor leukocyte infusions, nonmyeloablative conditioning and umbilical cord blood (UCB) transplantation.[2] As allogeneic HCT continues to increase, with more than 20,000 allogeneic transplantations performed annually worldwide, greater attention is given to improvements in supportive care, infectious prophylaxis, immuno-suppressive medications, and DNA-based tissue typing. Despite advances, graft-versus-host disease (GVHD) remains the most frequent and serious complication following allogeneic HCT and limits the broader application of this important therapy.[3] GVHD can be considered an exaggerated manifestation of a normal inflammatory mechanism in which donor lymphocytes encounter foreign antigens in a milieu that fosters inflammation. In the context of hematological malignancies, a delicate balance exists between the harmful consequences of GVHD and the beneficial effects incurred

Dr Choi is a St Baldrick's Career Development Scholar.

Dr Ferrara is an American Cancer Society Clinical Research Professor.

[a] Department of Pediatrics, Blood and Marrow Transplant Program, University of Michigan Medical School, 1500 E. Medical Center Drive, 6303 Comprehensive Cancer Center, Ann Arbor, MI 48109-5942, USA

[b] Department of Internal Medicine and Pediatrics, Blood and Marrow Transplant Program, University of Michigan Medical School, 1500 E. Medical Center Drive, 5303 Comprehensive Cancer Center, Ann Arbor, MI 48109-5941, USA

[c] Department of Internal Medicine and Pediatrics, Blood and Marrow Transplant Program, University of Michigan Medical School, 1500 E. Medical Center Drive, 6303 Comprehensive Cancer Center, Ann Arbor, MI 48109-5942, USA

* Corresponding author.

E-mail address: sungchoi@med.umich.edu (S.W. Choi).

when donor lymphocytes attack recipient malignant cells, a process referred to as the graft-versus-leukemia/tumor (GVL) effect. Given the increasing number of transplant recipients, there will be an increasing population of patients with GVHD. Recent advances in the understanding of the pathogenesis of GVHD have led to new approaches to its management, including using it to preserve the GVL effect following allogeneic transplant. This article reviews the important elements in the complex immunologic interactions involving cytokine networks, chemokine gradients, and the direct mediators of cellular cytotoxicity that cause clinical GVHD, and discusses the risk factors and strategies for management of GVHD.

ACUTE GVHD
Epidemiology and Risk Factors

In 1966, Billingham[4] formulated three requirements for the development of GVHD: the graft must contain immunologically competent cells; the recipient must express tissue antigens that are not present in the transplant donor; and the recipient must be incapable of mounting an effective response to eliminate the transplanted cells. It is now known that T cells are the immunologically competent cells, and when tissues containing T cells (blood products, bone marrow [BM], and solid organs) are transferred from one person to another who is unable to eliminate those cells, GVHD can develop.[5,6]

Allogeneic HCT is the most common setting for the development of GVHD, in which recipients receive immunoablative chemotherapy or radiation before hematopoietic cell infusion containing donor T cells. GVHD ultimately develops when donor T cells respond to recipient tissue antigens secondary to mismatches between major or minor histocompatibility antigens between the donor and recipient. The major histocompatibility complex (MHC) contains the genes that encode tissue antigens. In humans, the MHC region lies on the short arm of chromosome 6 and is called the human leukocyte antigen (HLA) region.[7] Class I HLA (A, B, and C) proteins are expressed on almost all nucleated cells of the body at varying densities. Class II (DR, DQ, and DP) proteins are primarily expressed on hematopoietic cells (B cells, dendritic cells, monocytes, and activated T cells), but their expression can be induced on many other cell types following inflammation or injury. High-resolution DNA typing of HLA genes with polymerase chain reaction (PCR)-based techniques has now largely replaced earlier methods. The incidence of GVHD is directly related to HLA disparity[8,9] and with more HLA mismatches, the likelihood of developing GVHD increases.[10,11] Recent data from the National Marrow Donor Program (NMDP) suggest that high-resolution matching for HLA-A, -B, -C, and -DRBI (8/8 match) maximizes post transplant survival.[12,13]

Despite HLA identity between a patient and donor, the incidence of acute GVHD ranges from 26% to 32% in recipients of sibling donor grafts, and 42% to 52% in recipients of unrelated donor grafts (Center for International Blood and Marrow Transplant Research [CIBMTR] Progress Report January–December 2008). The incidence is likely related to genetic differences that lie outside the HLA loci, or "minor" histocompatibility antigens (HA), which are immunogenic peptides derived from polymorphic proteins presented on the cell surface by MHC molecules.[14] Some minor HAs, such as HY and HA-3, are expressed on all tissues and are targets for GVHD and GVL, whereas other minor HAs, such as HA-1 and HA-2, are expressed abundantly on hematopoietic cells (including leukemic cells) and may induce a greater GVL effect with less GVHD.[14,15] However, the precise elucidation of most human minor antigens remains to be accomplished.[14,16]

The impact of donor and recipient polymorphisms in cytokine genes with critical roles in the classic "cytokine storm" of GVHD has been examined as a risk factor for GVHD.[17] Various polymorphic genes, including tumor necrosis factor α (TNF-α), interleukin 10 (IL-10), and interferon-γ (IFN-γ) variants, have been associated with GVHD, although not always.[18–20] There is no unequivocal evidence that polymorphic genes for cytokines or other proteins involved in innate immunity [21–24] sufficiently influence GVHD and transplant outcome to change clinical practice. Nonetheless, future strategies to identify the best possible transplant donor will likely incorporate HLA and non-HLA genetic factors.

In addition to genetic factors, other risk factors which have been associated with the development of GVHD include older donor and recipient age,[25–28] multiparous female donor,[28,29] advanced malignant condition at transplantation,[9,29] donor type,[28] and donor hematopoeitic cell source.[30–32] In the last decade, there has been a shift in clinical practice from the use of intraoperative harvested BM to granulocyte colony-stimulating factor mobilized peripheral blood stem cells (PBSC) as the donor hematopoietic cell source. However, definitive data demonstrating long-term advantages of PBSC rather than BM are lacking. One meta-analysis found that acute and chronic GVHD are more common following peripheral blood stem cell transplant (PBSCT) compared with bone marrow transplant (BMT) and indicated a trend toward decreased relapse rate following PBSCT.[31] The relative risk (RR) for acute GVHD after PBSCT was 1.16 (95% confidence interval [CI], 1.04–1.28) compared with BMT; the RR for chronic GVHD after PBSCT was 1.53 (95% CI, 1.25–2.05); and the RR for relapse after PBSCT was 0.81 (95% CI, 0.62–1.05). Thus, the survival benefit of PBSC versus BM remains in question. A large prospective, randomized, multicenter clinical trial of PBSC versus BM in unrelated donor transplantation conducted through the Blood and Marrow Transplant Clinical Trials Network (BMT CTN) has recently finished accrual.

For individuals without a suitable HLA-matched donor, UCB has become an alternative to BM or PBSC.[33–36] The incidence and severity of acute GVHD seem to be lower following UCB transplant than after HLA-matched marrow unrelated donor transplant, despite HLA disparities between the donor and recipient.[37,38] In an effort to meet the minimum cell dose required to ensure reliable engraftment, the simultaneous transplantation of 2 partially HLA-matched UCB units has been studied.[39] A recent report comparing transplantation with 2 partially HLA-matched UCB units versus a single unit demonstrated an increased incidence and earlier presentation of acute GVHD associated with the double UCB graft.[40]

Prevention

Prevention of acute GVHD is an integral component to the management of patients undergoing allogeneic HCT. The primary strategy employed is in the use of pharmacologic GVHD prophylaxis. The most widely used GVHD prophylaxis following full intensity conditioning includes a combination of a calcineurin inhibitor (eg, cyclosporine, tacrolimus) with methotrexate (MTX). This standard regimen was initially described in 1986[41] and since then several clinical trials have shown the superiority of this combination in reducing the incidence of GVHD and improving survival compared with either agent alone.[42–45] The calcineurin inhibitors cyclosporine and tacrolimus impede the function of the cytoplasmic enzyme calcineurin, which is critical to the activation of T cells. The most common side effects include hypomagnesemia, hyperkalemia, hypertension, and nephrotoxicity.[46] Large randomized studies comparing tacrolimus-MTX with cyclosporine-MTX have demonstrated a reduced incidence of grade II to IV acute GVHD with tacrolimus, but no overall survival advantage.[43,46]

Recently, sirolimus, a widely used immunosuppressant in solid organ transplantation,[47] has become attractive as a GVHD prophylactic agent because of the nonoverlapping toxicities with calcineurin inhibitors and the different mechanism of action. Sirolimus binds uniquely to FK binding protein 12 (FKBP12) and then complexes with mammalian Target of Rapamycin (mTOR).[48] Several studies have shown that the combination of sirolimus and tacrolimus has resulted in rapid engraftment, low incidence of acute GVHD, reduced transplant-related toxicity, and improved survival.[49] A prospective, randomized, multicenter trial is being conducted through the BMT CTN (protocol 0402) comparing sirolimus-tacrolimus versus tacrolimus-MTX following HLA-matched, related donor PBSCT.

A commonly used GVHD prophylaxis following reduced-intensity conditioning includes a combination of a calcineurin inhibitor (eg, cyclosporine, tacrolimus) with mycophenolate mofetil (MMF) instead of MTX. MMF, the prodrug of mycophenolic acid, selectively inhibits inosine monophosphate dehydrogenase, an enzyme critical to the de novo synthesis of guanosine nucleotide, which is needed for proliferation of T cells. In a prospective randomized trial, patients who received MMF as part of GVHD prophylaxis experienced significantly less severe mucositis and more rapid neutrophil engraftment than those who received MTX.[50] Although the optimal prophylaxis regimen following reduced-intensity HCT is not well established, MMF has been shown to be safe in this context.[51-55] MMF is also often preferred to MTX in UCB transplants because of its advantageous toxicity profile with respect to neutropenia and mucositis.

Many centers have previously attempted to decrease the risk of GVHD by ex vivo T cell depletion. Despite significant reductions in the incidence and severity of GVHD, T cell depletion has not achieved wide acceptance because of high rates of graft rejection, life-threatening infections, and leukemia relapse.[56-58] In vivo T cell depletion has also been widely studied using alemtuzumab, a monoclonal antibody specific for CD52 antigen expressed abundantly on the surface of normal and malignant lymphocytes,[59,60] or antithymocyte globulin (ATG), a polyclonal antibody mixture of either horse or rabbit origin directed against multiple epitopes of human T cells.[61] These approaches are associated with significant reduction in acute GVHD, but at the cost of impaired immune reconstitution and increased risk of leukemia relapse. Thus, the focus of most prevention strategies remains pharmacologic manipulation of T cells following transplant.

Pathophysiology

Acute GVHD is mediated by donor lymphocytes infused into the recipient, in whom they encounter profoundly damaged tissues from the effects of the underlying disease, prior infections, and the transplant conditioning regimen. The allogeneic donor cells encounter a foreign environment that has been altered to promote the activation and proliferation of inflammatory cells. Thus, acute GVHD reflects an exaggerated response of the normal inflammatory mechanisms that involves donor T cells and multiple innate and adaptive cells and mediators. Three sequential phases can be conceptualized to illustrate the complex cellular interactions and inflammatory cascades that ultimately evolve to acute GVHD: (1) activation of antigen-presenting cells (APCs); (2) donor T cell activation, proliferation, differentiation and migration; and (3) target tissue destruction.[62]

Phase 1: activation of APCs

In the first phase, APCs are activated by the underlying disease and the HCT conditioning regimen.[63] Animal models [63,64] and clinical HCT [65] have supported the observation that increased risk of GVHD is associated with intensive conditioning regimens that contribute to extensive tissue injury and subsequent release of inflammatory cytokines. Damage to host tissues leads to the secretion of proinflammatory cytokines, such as TNF-α and IL-1, and chemokines, such as CCL2-5 and CXCL9-11, thereby producing increased expression of adhesion molecules, MHC antigens and costimulatory molecules on host APCs. For example, increase of plasma TNF-α receptor 1 levels, a surrogate marker for TNF-α, at 1 week after HCT strongly correlates with the later development of GVHD.[66] Systemic translocation of immunostimulatory microbial products, such as lipopolysaccharide (LPS), as a result of damage to the gastrointestinal (GI) tract induced by the conditioning regimen, enhances the activation of host APCs.[67,68] The initial site of interaction between activated APCs and donor T cells is likely the secondary lymphoid tissue in the GI tract.[69] Different distinct subsets of APCs, including host and donor type APCs,[68,70,71] dendritic cells,[72,73] Langerhans cells,[74] and monocytes/macrophages,[75] have been implicated in this phase. However, the relative contributions of these various APCs remain to be elucidated. The intensity of the conditioning regimen and the degree of tissue injury seem to be associated with the risk of GVHD. Reduced intensity conditioning regimens have thus become more widely employed in an effort to reduce acute GVHD by decreasing the damage to host tissues.[65,76]

Phase 2: donor T cell activation

Donor T cell activation, proliferation, differentiation, and migration in response to primed APCs occur during the second phase of acute GVHD. The T cell receptors (TCR) of donor T cells recognize alloantigens on host and donor type APCs that are present in secondary lymphoid organs.[77,78] During direct presentation, donor T cells recognize either the peptide bound to host MHC molecules, or the foreign MHC molecules themselves.[79] During indirect presentation, donor T cells respond to the peptides generated by degradation of the host MHC molecules that are presented on donor-derived MHC.[80]

Following antigen recognition, signaling through the TCR induces a conformational change in adhesion molecules, resulting in high affinity binding to the APC.[81] The complex interaction between T cell costimulatory molecules and their ligands on APCs facilitates full T cell activation. Many T cell costimulatory molecules display unique and overlapping functions.[82] Receptors of the B7 family and the TNF family play especially critical roles in GVHD, and are known to deliver positive and negative signals to T cells.[83] Blockade of costimulatory and inhibitory pathways can reduce acute GVHD in murine models, but this approach has not yet been tested in clinical trials.[2]

Murine studies have shown that control of alloreactive responses responsible for GVHD depends at least in part on CD4+ CD25+ regulatory T cells. Studies in mice suggest that regulatory T cells added to donor grafts can prevent or delay GVHD.[84] However, the role of regulatory T cells in clinical allogeneic HCT has not been well established, in part because of the lack of clear identification of human regulatory T cell phenotype. In contrast to murine studies, more severe acute GVHD developed clinically when donor grafts contained larger numbers of donor CD4+ CD25+ T cells.[85] One recent study found that HCT recipients with higher absolute numbers of FOXP3+ CD4+ T cells were associated with a reduced risk of developing GVHD.[86] However, FOXP3 expression in humans is not specific for regulatory T cell phenotype,[87] and improved techniques to identify and expand regulatory T cells are required for its wider application in clinical BMT.

Several intracellular biochemical pathways are rapidly amplified following T cell activation. Activated T cells secrete cytokines that are generally classified as Th1 (IFN-γ,

IL-2 and TNF-α) or Th2 (IL-4, IL-5, IL-10, and IL-13) and Th17. Although Th1 cytokines induce GVHD efficiently, the balance of Th1 and Th2 cytokines is important in the immunopathogenesis of GVHD, but remains incompletely understood.[88] TNF-α, already discussed as an inducer of APC activation in phase I, functions to amplify T cell activation and proliferation in this second phase of GVHD. IL-2 production is also integral in this early development of acute GVHD,[89] and remains the principal target of many current clinical therapeutic and prophylactic approaches to GVHD, such as cyclosporine, tacrolimus, and monoclonal antibodies against IL-2 and its receptor.[44] However, recent data suggest that regulatory T cell function is dependent on the presence of calcineurin-dependent IL-2, and that interference with IL-2 may possibly antagonize the induction of tolerance.[90]

IFN-γ is a cytokine with diverse effects in vivo that can amplify and suppress acute GVHD. With regards to amplification, IFN-γ increases the expression of molecules such as chemokine receptors, MHC proteins, and adhesion molecules. IFN-γ also sensitizes monocytes and macrophages to stimuli such as LPS, thereby accelerating intracellular cascades in response to these stimuli.[88] IFN-γ may also amplify GVHD by directly damaging target cells in the GI tract and in the skin while conversely inducing nitric oxide-mediated immunosuppression.[91] IFN-γ itself can prevent experimental GVHD by hastening the apoptosis of activated donor T cells.[92] Thus, this complexity makes it a challenging target with respect to therapeutic intervention.

IL-10 can suppress the expression of proinflammatory cytokines, chemokines, and adhesion molecules, and antigen-presenting and costimulatory molecules in monocytes/macrophages, neutrophils, and T cells.[93] Recent clinical data suggest that genetic polymorphism in the IL-10 promoter region of the recipient has a significant impact on the risk of developing acute GVHD.[94] Increased IL-10 production by recipient cells stimulated ex vivo has been associated with a reduced risk of acute GVHD.[95] Experimental data have also demonstrated that transforming growth factor β (TGF-β), another suppressive cytokine, attenuates acute GVHD, but may lead to chronic GVHD.[96] Thus multiple cytokines are important in GVHD pathogenesis and regulation. Furthermore, the timing and duration of cytokine expression may be a critical factor determining the induction of the GVH reaction, and cytokine dysregulation could potentially contribute to the severity of acute GVHD.[62]

Phase 3: cellular and inflammatory effector phase

A complex cascade of cellular and inflammatory mediators occurs during the effector phase of acute GVHD. These mediators synergize to amplify local tissue injury and damage target tissues. As such, the effector phase of GVHD involves aspects of the innate and adaptive immune response and interactions with the proinflammatory cells and cytokines generated during phase 1 and 2.

Cellular effectors Cytotoxic T cells are the major cellular effectors of acute GVHD and lyse target cells using principally the Fas/Fas ligand (FasL) and the perforin/granzyme pathways.[97] The Fas-FasL pathway seems to predominate in hepatic GVHD whereas the perforin/granzyme pathways are more important in the GI tract and skin.[2] The "danger" signals generated in phase 1, augmented by the expression of costimulatory molecules in phase 2, induce the production of chemokines. The migration of donor T cells from lymphoid tissues to the target organs in which damage occurs is directed by these chemokine gradients and adhesion molecules such as L-selectin and $\alpha_L\beta_2$ integrin. The upregulation of chemokines, such as CCL2, CCL3, CCL4, CCL5, CXCL9, CXCL10, and CXCL11 in GVHD target organs (skin, liver, and gut), play primary roles in this homing process.[98] Furthermore, integrin receptors, which are regulated by chemokines, mediate many adhesive interactions that are critical for successful T cell migration.[99]

Inflammatory effectors The secretion of inflammatory cytokines, such as TNF-α or IL-1 also results in GVHD target organ injury. The secretion signal may be provided through toll-like receptors (TLRs) by LPS and other microbial products that have leaked through damaged intestinal mucosa by the conditioning regimen in phase 1.[100] TNF-α is produced by donor and host cells and is a critical component of GVHD pathophysiology. TNF-α can (1) activate APCs and enhance alloantigen presentation, (2) recruit effector cells to target organs through the induction of inflammatory chemokines, and (3) directly cause tissue damage via apoptosis and necrosis. IL-1 is also involved in the pathogenesis of acute GVHD.[17] Its secretion occurs predominantly in the spleen and skin during the effector phase of experimental GVHD.[101] Increased expression of mononuclear IL-1 mRNA has been associated with the development of GVHD.[102] However, the blockade of IL-1 using recombinant human IL-1 receptor antagonist in patients undergoing HCT did not reduce the risk of GVHD.[103]

Clinical Features

The three main organs involved in acute GVHD are the skin, liver, or GI tract. GVHD presents clinically in an acute or chronic form. Historically, the acute and chronic forms were arbitrarily defined based on the timeframe post transplant (less than or more than 100 days, respectively).[104] However, current consensus is that clinical manifestations guide whether the signs and symptoms of GVHD are acute, chronic, or an overlap syndrome (wherein diagnostic or distinctive features of acute and chronic GVHD appear together).[105]

The extent (stage) of involvement of the three principal target organs determines the overall severity (grade) of acute GVHD (**Table 1**).[106] The overall grades are classified as I (mild), II (moderate), III (severe), and IV (very severe). A poor prognosis is associated with severe grade III or IV GVHD, with 25% and 5% overall survival, respectively.[107]

Skin is generally the first and most commonly affected organ.[104] The presentation of skin involvement generally coincides with donor cell engraftment and is characterized by an erythematous, maculopapular rash that is often pruritic. In severe cases the skin may blister and ulcerate.[108] The pathognomonic histopathologic finding is apoptosis at the base of epidermal rete ridges. Other features include dyskeratosis, exocytosis of lymphocytes, satellite lymphocytes adjacent to dyskeratotic epidermal keratinocytes, and a perivascular lymphocytic infiltration in the dermis.[1,109]

Liver GVHD can be a challenging diagnosis. The initial feature typically includes the development of jaundice or an increase in the alkaline phosphatase and bilirubin; hepatomegaly may be noted. However, it is often difficult to distinguish from other causes of liver dysfunction following allogeneic HCT, such as drug toxicity, venoocclusive disease, opportunistic (bacterial, viral, and fungal) infections, total parenteral nutrition, acalculous cholecystitis, and iron overload, because of the overlapping patterns of clinical history, physical examination, and laboratory and imaging data. Thus, a biopsy is often required to confirm the diagnosis of liver GVHD.[110] The histologic features are endothelialitis, lymphocytic infiltration of the portal areas, pericholangitis, and bile duct destruction.[111] However, the increased risk of bleeding associated with thrombocytopenia in the immediate post transplant period can preclude obtaining a biopsy. As such, the diagnosis of liver GVHD is often a clinical diagnosis of exclusion.

GI tract involvement of acute GVHD may present as nausea, vomiting, anorexia, diarrhea, or abdominal pain. It is a panintestinal process with focal lesions of varying

Table 1
Acute GVHD grading criteria

Stage	Skin	Liver (Bilirubin)	GI Tract (Stool Output/d)
0	No GVHD rash	<2 mg/dL	Adult: <500 mL/d Child: <10 mL kg/d
1	Maculopapular rash <25% BSA	2–3 mg/dL	Adult: 500–999 mL/d Child: 10–19.9 mL/kg/d or persistent nausea, vomiting, or anorexia, with a positive upper GI biopsy
2	Maculopapular rash 25%–50% BSA	3.1–6 mg/dL	Adult: 1000–1500 mL/d Child: 20–30 mL/kg/d
3	Maculopapular rash >50% BSA	6.1–15 mg/dL	Adult: >1500 mL/d Child: >30 mL/kg/d
4	Generalized erythroderma with bullous formation	>15 mg/dL	Severe abdominal pain with or without ileus

Overall clinical grade: grade 0, no stage 1–4 of any organ; 1, stage 1–2 skin rash and no liver or GI involvement; 2, stage 3 skin rash, or stage 1 liver involvement, or stage 1 GI involvement; 3, stage 0–3 skin rash, with stage 2–3 liver involvement, or stage 2–3 GI involvement; 4, stage 4 skin rash, liver, or GI involvement.

The standard GVHD grading criteria were developed by Glucksberg in 1974. (*Data from* Glucksberg H, Storb R, Fefer A, et al. Clinical manifestations of graft-versus-host disease in human recipients of marrow from HL-A-matched sibling donors. Transplantation 1974;18(4):295–304) and then revised at the 1994 Consensus Conference in Keystone. (*Data from* Pzrepiorka D, Weisdorf D, Martin P, et al. Consensus conference on acute GVHD grading. Bone Marrow Transpl 1995;15:825–8.) The grading system did not initially take into consideration the staging of the GI tract for pediatric patients. However, most pediatric centers have adopted the modified Glucksberg grading scale and adjusted the staging of the GI tract to be based on volume per kg of body weight.

Abbreviation: BSA, body surface area.

intensity. Gastric involvement causes postprandial vomiting that is not always preceded by nausea. The diarrhea of GVHD is secretory and may be accompanied by significant GI bleeding as a result of mucosal ulceration, which is a prognostic factor for poor outcome.[112] In advanced disease, diffuse, severe abdominal pain and distension are accompanied by voluminous diarrhea. The histologic features include patchy ulcerations, apoptotic bodies in the base of crypts, crypt abscesses, and loss and flattening of the epithelium surface.[113]

Diagnostic Approach

The diagnosis of acute GVHD is based entirely on clinical criteria that can be confirmed by biopsy of one of the three target organs. Laboratory data or imaging studies are also useful tests in the diagnostic approach to GVHD. However, a major challenge with the diagnosis is the absence of laboratory tests that can reliably predict or screen for the condition before its onset: that can establish a diagnosis in real time; that can distinguish it from other conditions that present with similar symptoms, such as infection; or that can stratify patients according to response to therapy. Thus, experimental blood tests with predictive value for GVHD such as a 4-biomarker panel[114,115] may ultimately be useful to further identify high-risk groups and their outcomes (**Fig. 1**). These biomarkers could result in immunosuppressive treatment schemas tailored to patients in several risk groups.

A

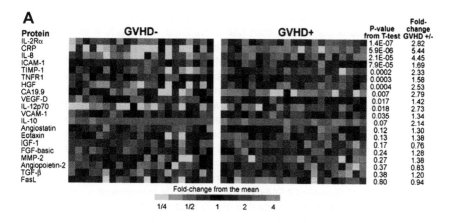

Protein	P-value from T-test	Fold-change GVHD +/-
IL-2Rα	1.4E-07	2.82
CRP	5.9E-06	5.44
IL-8	2.1E-05	4.45
ICAM-1	7.9E-05	1.69
TIMP-1	0.0002	2.33
TNFR1	0.0003	1.58
HGF	0.0004	2.53
CA19.9	0.007	2.79
VEGF-D	0.017	1.42
IL-12p70	0.018	2.73
VCAM-1	0.035	1.34
IL-10	0.07	2.14
Angiostatin	0.12	1.30
Eotaxin	0.13	1.38
IGF-1	0.17	0.76
FGF-basic	0.24	1.28
MMP-2	0.27	1.38
Angiopoietin-2	0.37	0.83
TGF-β	0.38	1.20
FasL	0.80	0.94

B

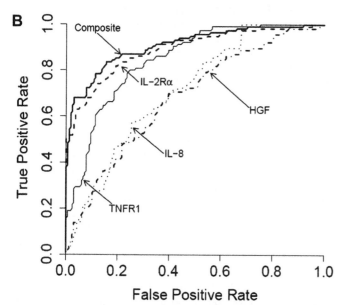

Fig. 1. From discovery to validation of plasma biomarkers of acute GVHD. (*A*) The heatmap of proteins levels measured sequential enzyme-linked immunosorbent assay in the discovery set samples. Samples from 21 GVHD− patients (*left*) and 21 GVHD+ patients (*right*) are represented. Eleven proteins gave a *P* value for differences between GVHD+ and GVHD− patient plasma <0.05. (*B*) The receiver-operating characteristic (ROC) curves of 4 individual discriminator proteins and the composite panel in the training set. Individual ROC curves for IL-2Ra, TNFR1, human growth factor, and IL-8 and the composite panel. (*From* Paczesny S, Krijanovski OI, Braun TM, et al. A biomarker panel for acute graft-versus-host disease. Blood 2009;113(2):273–8; with permission.)

Treatment

Despite routine treatment with calcineurin-based prophylaxis, GVHD remains a major complication of allogeneic HCT. The most important predictor of long-term survival in patients with acute GVHD is the primary response to the first line of treatment.[116] Many centers treat mild skin GVHD (grade I) with topical corticosteroids alone, but for more severe skin GVHD or visceral GVHD involvement (grade II or greater), systemic corticosteroids are the mainstay of therapy, typically starting at 1 to 2 mg/kg/d. Durable responses occur in less than half of patients with grade II to IV GVHD,[117] and with increasing severity of the disease, the likelihood of response decreases.[104] Treatment with high-dose steroids often continues for 7 days or more, with a gradual dose reduction depending on the clinical response. In a recent retrospective analysis, low-dose (1 mg/kg/d) versus high-dose (2 mg/kg/d) prednisone was compared for initial treatment of acute GVHD. In patients with grades I to II GVHD, the nonrelapse mortality and overall survival were similar between regimens, with a reduced risk of invasive fungal infections and shorter hospitalizations in the low-dose prednisone group. The number of patients with grades III to IV at onset was too few to draw any significant conclusions.

In addition to topical corticosteroid therapy for skin GVHD, nonabsorbed steroid therapy is commonly used in GI GVHD. Oral budesonide in combination with systemic corticosteroids in patients with grade II or higher acute GI GVHD has shown complete responses in 77% of patients compared with 32% of historical controls.[118] In a more recent randomized, placebo-controlled trial of oral beclomethasone for GI GVHD, oral beclomethasone dipropionate (BDP) reduced GVHD flares following a prednisone taper and resulted in superior survival at 1 year post transplant.[119] Intraarterial administration of steroids for GI and hepatic GVHD has also been attempted to deliver steroids directly to the target organ.[120]

Prolonged therapy with steroids invariably increases the risk of patients developing muscle weakness and wasting, avascular necrosis, compression fractures, hypertension, hyperglycemia, behavior disturbances, and life-threatening infections. Furthermore, the optimal dose and duration of high-dose steroids, and the choice and timing of when to institute second therapy, remain unclear.[121] Thus, the management of a patient who develops steroid-refractory acute GVHD is challenging. Generally, steroid-refractoriness is defined as disease progression or lack of response following 3 to 7 days of systemic therapy with corticosteroids and a calcineurin inhibitor. Once steroid-refractory GVHD develops, various agents may be used, and there is currently no standard approach practiced uniformly by the transplant community.

Table 2 summarizes the various drugs that have been studied in addition to steroids for treatment of acute GVHD. Among the agents discussed, MMF, etanercept, denileukin diftitox and pentostatin were most recently studied in a clinical investigation through the BMT CTN (study 0302). In this phase II, randomized trial of 180 patients with newly diagnosed acute GVHD, patients were treated with standard corticosteroids plus one of the four agents. MMF produced the best results with regards to toxicity profile, response, survival, incidence of chronic GVHD, and infections.[122] A randomized phase III study to validate these findings is being planned.

Extracorporeal photopheresis (ECP) is increasingly used in the management of acute and chronic GVHD in an effort to minimize corticosteroid exposure. During ECP, the patient's peripheral blood mononuclear cells are exposed to photo-activated 8-methoxypsoralen (8-MOP) and ultraviolet A radiation, which covalently binds and cross-links DNA, and then returned to the patient. Experimental studies in humans and mice suggest ECP induces apoptosis of the mononuclear cells and increases the number of regulatory T cells.[123,124] A phase II study of steroid-refractory GVHD showed complete response rates of 60%, with overall survival of 59% at 4 years.[125] These data are similar to other studies that have demonstrated complete response rates between 52% and 83%.[126–128]

Mesenchymal stromal cell infusion is another nonpharmacologic approach, but little is known about its mechanism of action. In vitro, mesenchymal stromal cells have various effects on immune cells, including T cells, APCs, natural killer cells, and B

Table 2
Selected studies of novel agents as secondary or first-line therapy in acute GVHD

Novel Therapy	Type of Trial	Type of Treatment	Sample Size	Overall Response at 4 Weeks (%)	Survival at 3-6 Months (%)	Study	References
Denileukin diftitox	Phase I	Steroid refractory	30	71	33	Ho et al	146
Denileukin diftitox	Phase II	Steroid refractory	22	41	ND	Shaughnessy et al	147
Denileukin diftitox	Phase II randomized	Initial therapy	47	60	49	Alousi et al	122
Etanercept	Phase II	Initial therapy	61	69	69	Levine et al	148
Etanercept	Phase II randomized	Initial therapy	46	48	56	Alousi et al	122
Pentostatin	Phase I	Steroid refractory	23	78	ND	Bolanos-Meade et al	149
Pentostatin	Phase II randomized	Initial therapy	42	62	52	Alousi et al	122
MMF	Phase I/II	Steroid refractory	48	72	78	Basara et al	150
MMF	Phase I/II	Steroid refractory	10	60	70	Krejci et al	151
MMF	Phase I/II	Steroid refractory	6	67	64	Takami et al	152
MMF	Phase II randomized	Initial therapy	45	78	64	Alousi et al	122
Sirolimus	Phase I/II	Steroid refractory	21	57	28	Benito et al	153
BDP	Phase II randomized	Initial therapy	129	71	87	Hockenbery et al	119
ECP	Phase II	Steroid refractory	59	68	ND	Greinix et al	125
ECP	Phase II	Steroid refractory	23	52	48	Perfetti et al	126
ECP	Phase II	Steroid refractory	41 (children)	73	100	Calore et al	127
ECP	Phase II	Steroid refractory	15 (children)	0 (for grade IV GVHD)	ND	Berger et al	128
MSC	Phase II	steroid refractory	55	71	ND	Le Blanc et al	130
MSC	Phase II	Steroid refractory	13	15	31	von Bonin et al	154
Alefacept	Phase I	Steroid refractory	16	75	ND	Shapira et al	155

Abbreviations: ECP, extracorporeal photopheresis; MSC, mesenchymal stromal cell; ND, not determined.

cells. In phase I and II trials, HLA-identical mesenchymal stromal cells expanded ex vivo have been infused to promote hematopoietic recovery after autologous and allogeneic HCT.[129,130] In a phase II study, mesenchymal stem cells were used for the treatment of corticosteroid-resistant, severe, acute GVHD.[130] Thirty-nine of 55 patients with corticosteroid-resistant, severe, acute GVHD responded to treatment with mesenchymal stem cells. In those who achieved a complete response, survival was significantly higher and transplant-related mortality was lower compared with those with partial or no response. No major toxicities were observed, and treatment with mesenchymal stem cells seemed to be safe. This therapy may be a promising treatment of corticosteroid-refractory acute GVHD, but further investigation is required.

CHRONIC GVHD
Epidemiology and Risk Factors

Chronic GVHD is the major cause of late nonrelapse death following allogeneic HCT,[131] and is associated with decreased quality of life and impaired physical and functional status.[132] It remains the most common problem in long-term survivors. However, chronic GVHD has been associated with beneficial GVL/GVT effects.[133] The median time of diagnosis of chronic GVHD is 4.5 months after HLA-identical sibling transplantation and 4 months after unrelated donor transplantation.[134] The incidence of chronic GVHD has been increasing with the wider availability of PBSC and the increased age of transplant recipients. The development of chronic GVHD ranges from 30% in recipients of fully histocompatible sibling donor transplants to 60% to 70% in recipients of mismatched hematopoietic cells or hematopoietic cells from an unrelated donor. Other factors that likely increase the development of chronic GVHD include prior acute GVHD, older recipient age, female donor (multiparous, in particular) with a male recipient, and use of PBSC.[132]

Prevention and Pathophysiology

Although prevention of acute GVHD has improved during the past three decades, no effective prophylaxis regimen exists for chronic GVHD. Management of chronic GVHD is guided by a multidisciplinary approach to treatment, including recent adjustment of immunosuppressive medications and aggressive supportive care.

Understanding of the pathophysiology of chronic GVHD is not so advanced as that of acute GVHD. Chronic GVHD is a complex, multisystem disorder with myriad manifestations that involves many different organs (see later discussion). It is characterized by immune dysregulation, immunodeficiency, impaired organ function, and decreased survival.[135] Alloreactive T cells have been implicated in the pathogenesis; however, the precise role of specific T cell subsets, autoantigens, alloantigens, and B cells, and interactions of chemokines and cytokines has not been fully elucidated. The clinical manifestations of chronic GVHD are often similar to an autoimmune process, suggesting similar pathophysiology.

Clinical Features

The diagnosis of chronic GVHD is based on specific signs, degree of organ involvement (mild, moderate, severe), laboratory data, or histopathologic confirmation rather than time of onset post transplant (ie, >100 days). Historically, a classification of "limited" (localized skin involvement with or without limited hepatic dysfunction) versus "extensive" (generalized skin involvement or limited disease plus eye, oral, liver, or other target organ involvement) was the most commonly adopted staging system.[136] However, new consensus criteria for the diagnosis and staging of chronic GVHD have been proposed by the National Institutes of Health (NIH) Consensus Development Project (**Table 3**).[105] Chronic GVHD may present as acute GVHD merging into chronic (progressive type), develop following a period of resolution from acute GVHD (quiescent or interrupted type), or occur de novo. An overlap syndrome includes clinical features in which diagnostic or distinctive features of chronic GVHD and acute GVHD appear together. Specific signs and symptoms, including erythematous skin rash, nausea, vomiting, diarrhea, and liver dysfunction are shared between the two.

Diagnostic Approach

The potential clinical manifestations of chronic GVHD are many and varied, involving multiple organs and sites. At least one distinctive manifestation for chronic GVHD is required to diagnose chronic GVHD, such as oral or vaginal lichenoid findings, ocular sicca, skin dyspigmentation, scleroderma, or bronchiolitis obliterans. Biopsies or other diagnostic tests (eg, laboratory tests, radiographic tests, or pulmonary tests) are recommended to confirm the diagnosis of chronic GVHD. Definitive diagnosis of chronic GVHD requires excluding other possible diagnoses such as infection, drug effects, malignancies, and residual postinflammatory damage and scarring.

Treatment

Definitive treatment of chronic GVHD, including the implementation and withdrawal of specific therapies, remains elusive. The prior use of prophylaxis agents or the history of therapies used in acute GVHD ultimately affects the choice of treatment of chronic GVHD, as do the specific patient characteristics and preferences of the treating physician and center. Generally, treatment of chronic GVHD is less intense and less aggressive than that used for acute GVHD, but may require a prolonged duration of multimodal immunosuppressive therapy. The most widely used first-line therapy for patients with chronic GVHD is a combination of systemic corticosteroids and a calcineurin inhibitor. The recently published NIH guidelines recommend this treatment if three or more organs are involved or any single organ has a severity score of more than 2.[105] The NIH Working Group defines failure of initial therapy or requirement of additional secondary therapy as follows: (1) progression of chronic GVHD despite optimal first-line therapy (including >1 mg/kg/d of prednisolone for 2 weeks), or (2) no improvement after 4 to 8 weeks of sustained therapy, or (3) inability to taper corticosteroid dose.[105]

Chronic immunosuppressants, especially those containing steroids, are toxic and often result in life-threatening infectious complications. Many second-line therapies for chronic GVHD have been studied, but none has achieved widespread acceptance. Agents studied in chronic GVHD include ECP, MMF, and rituximab. ECP has demonstrated significant response rates in high-risk chronic GVHD patients, particularly in the skin, liver, oral mucosa, eye, and lung.[137] However, the response of chronic GVHD to treatment is often unpredictable, and mixed responses in different organs can occur in the same patient. MMF showed initial promise, but in a multicenter placebo-controlled randomized trial, the addition of MMF to the initial systemic treatment regimen for chronic GVHD did not show any benefit.[138] In small phase II trials, rituximab, an anti-CD20 chimeric monoclonal antibody, has demonstrated an overall response rate of 65% to 70% for its use in refractory chronic GVHD.[139,140] More recently, it has been shown that patients with fibrotic, chronic GVHD have antibodies activating the platelet-derived growth factor receptor pathway.[141] In this light, a pilot

Table 3
Signs and symptoms of chronic GVHD

Organ or Site	Diagnostic (Sufficient to Establish the Diagnosis of Chronic GVHD)	Distinctive (Seen in Chronic GVHD, but Insufficient Alone to Establish a Diagnosis of Chronic GVHD)	Other Features[a]	Common (Seen with Acute and Chronic GVHD)
Skin	Poikiloderma Lichen planus-like features Morphea-like features Lichen sclerosus-like features	Depigmentation	Sweat impairment Ichthyosis Keratosis pilaris Hypopigmentation Hyperpigmentation	Erythema Maculopapular rash Pruritis
Nails		Dystrophy Longitudinal ridging, splitting, or brittle features Onycholysis Pterygium unguis Nail loss (usually symmetric; affects most nails)[b]		
Scalp and body hair		New onset of scarring or nonscarring scallop alopecia (after recovery from chemoradiotherapy) Scaling, papulosquamous lesions	Thinning scalp hair, typically patchy, coarse, or dull (not explained by endocrine or other causes) Premature gray hair	

Mouth	Lichen-type features Hyperkeratotic plaques Restriction of mouth opening from sclerosis	Xerostomia Mucocele Mucosal atrophy Pseudomembranes[b] Ulcers[b]	Gingivitis Mucositis Erythema Pain
Eyes		New onset dry, gritty, or painful eyes[c] Cicatricial conjunctivitis Keratoconjunctivitis sicca[c] Confluent areas of punctate keratopathy	Photophobia Periorbital hyperpigmentation Blepharitis (erythema of the eyelids with edema)
Genitalia	Lichen planus-like features Vaginal scarring or stenosis	Erosions[b] Fissures[b] Ulcers[b]	
GI tract	Esophageal web Strictures of stenosis in the upper to mid-third of the esophagus[b]	Exocrine pancreatic insufficiency	Anorexia Nausea Vomiting Diarrhea Weight loss Failure to thrive (infants and children) Total bilirubin, alkaline phosphatase more than twice upper limit of normal[b] ALT or AST more than twice upper limit of normal[b]

(continued on next page)

Table 3
(continued)

Organ or Site	Diagnostic (Sufficient to Establish the Diagnosis of Chronic GVHD)	Distinctive (Seen in Chronic GVHD, but Insufficient Alone to Establish a Diagnosis of Chronic GVHD)	Other Features[a]	Common (Seen with Acute and Chronic GVHD)
Lung	Bronchiolitis obliterans diagnosed with lung biopsy	Bronchiolitis obliterans diagnosed with PFTs and radiology[c]		BOOP
Muscles, fascia, joints	Fasciitis Joint stiffness or contractures secondary to sclerosis	Myositis of polymyositis[c]	Edema Muscle cramps Arthralgia or arthritis	
Hematopoietic and immune			Thrombocytopenia Eosinophilia Lymphopenia Hypo- or hypergammaglobulinemia Autoantibodies (AIGA and ITP)	
Other			Pericardial or pleural effusions Ascites Peripheral neuropathy Nephrotic syndrome Myasthema gravis Cardiac conduction abnormality or cardiomyopathy	

Abbreviations: AIGA, autoimmune hemolytic anemia; ALT, alanine aminotransferase; AST, aspartate aminotransferase; BOOP, bronchiolitis obliterans-organizing pneumonia; ITP, idiopathic thrombocytopenic purpura; PFTs, pulmonary function tests.

[a] Can be acknowledged as part of the chronic GVHD symptomatology if the diagnosis is confirmed.

[b] In all cases, infection, drug effects, malignancy, or other causes must be excluded.

[c] Diagnosis of chronic GVHD required biopsy or radiology confirmation (or Schirmer test for eyes).

Reproduced from Filipovich AH, Weisdorf D, Pavletic S, et al. National Institutes of Health consensus development project on criteria for clinical trials in chronic graft-versus-host disease: I. Diagnosis and staging working group report. Biol Blood Marrow Transplant 2005;11(12):945–56; with permission.

study in 19 patients with refractory chronic GVHD investigated imatinib, which inhibits this pathway. At 6 months, the overall response rate was 79%, with 7 complete remissions and 8 partial remissions.[142] These promising results deserve larger exploration and longer study.

Supportive Care in the Management of GVHD Patients

Supportive care and routine monitoring are critical in the management of chronic GVHD. Early recognition of high-risk features (such as thrombocytopenia, progressive onset chronic GVHD, extensive skin involvement with sclerodermatous features, and multiorgan involvement) and appropriate early intervention are important.[105] The Ancillary Therapy and Supportive Care Working Group, as part of the 2005 NIH-sponsored Consensus Conference in chronic GVHD, recently established guidelines for ancillary and supportive care therapies.[137] Routine interval history, physical examination with assessment of symptoms, review of medications, laboratory monitoring (complete blood cell counts with differential, chemistry panel to assess kidney and liver functions, drug monitoring, IgG levels, lipid profiles, and endocrine evaluations to assess thyroid function, calcium, and vitamin D levels) and the consultation of appropriate subspecialists should be performed. It is important that transplant physicians and primary hematologists recognize the increased incidence of second malignancies in transplant recipients, particularly squamous cell carcinoma in chronic GVHD patients.[143] Furthermore, specific attention to the surveillance of infection prophylaxis (anti-bacterial, -viral, and -fungal), vaccinations, general hygiene, physical therapy, nutritional status, pain control, and monitoring of drug-drug interactions and the associated drug-related side effects, is required. There is little supporting evidence for the routine use of intravenous immunoglobulin as prophylaxis,[144] but patients should receive routine antibiotic prophylaxis (penicillin or its equivalent) because of the increased risk of streptococcal sepsis.[145] The sites of any indwelling catheter should be assessed regularly. Early recognition of signs or symptoms of septic shock requires prompt evaluation with blood cultures and initiation of broad spectrum antibiotics.

Future Directions

The population of patients with GVHD has steadily grown as the number of allogeneic transplantations being performed annually has increased. Newer treatment approaches and wider availability of supportive care and ancillary therapies have led to improved survival. Despite these recent advances, however, GVHD remains a leading cause of morbidity and mortality in survivors of allogeneic transplantation. Novel approaches to GVHD are thus urgently needed. In this light, it is important to recognize that the management of patients with GVHD is complex and requires a multidisciplinary approach. A major barrier to current therapies is life-threatening infectious complications caused by broad nonspecific immune suppression. Future strategies are likely to include modulation of cell types that play key roles in the GVHD process, including regulatory T cells, dendritic cells, natural killer T cells, and B cells. As such, targeted therapies are preferable to preserve the beneficial antitumor effect while eliminating the debilitating consequences of GVHD. Identification of biomarkers for GVHD with diagnostic and prognostic significance may further clarify groups of patients at highest risk and eventually improve the management of GVHD.

REFERENCES

1. Ferrara JL, Deeg HJ. Graft-versus-host disease. N Engl J Med 1991;324(10): 667–74.
2. Welniak LA, Blazar BR, Murphy WJ. Immunobiology of allogeneic hematopoietic stem cell transplantation. Annu Rev Immunol 2007;25:139–70.
3. Reddy P, Arora M, Guimond M, et al. GVHD: a continuing barrier to the safety of allogeneic transplantation. Biol Blood Marrow Transplant 2008;15(Suppl 1): 162–8.
4. Billingham RE. The biology of graft-versus-host reactions. Harvey Lect 1966;62: 21–78.
5. Korngold R, Sprent J. Purified T cell subsets and lethal graft-versus-host disease in mice. In: Gale RP, Champlin R, editors. Progress in bone marrow transplant. New York: Alan R. Liss, Inc; 1987. p. 213–8.
6. Kernan NA, Collins NH, Juliano LL, et al. Clonable T lymphocytes in T cell-depleted bone marrow transplants correlate with development of graft-v-host disease. Blood 1986;68(3):770–3.
7. Erlich HA, Opelz G, Hansen J. HLA DNA typing and transplantation. Immunity 2001;14(4):347–56.
8. Loiseau P, Busson M, Balere ML, et al. HLA Association with hematopoietic stem cell transplantation outcome: the number of mismatches at HLA-A, -B, -C, -DRB1, or -DQB1 is strongly associated with overall survival. Biol Blood Marrow Transplant 2007;13(8):965–74.
9. Hahn T, McCarthy PL Jr, Zhang MJ, et al. Risk factors for acute graft-versus-host disease after human leukocyte antigen-identical sibling transplants for adults with leukemia. J Clin Oncol 2008;26(35):5728–34.
10. Kernan NA, Bartsch G, Ash RC, et al. Analysis of 462 transplantations from unre-lated donors facilitated by the National Marrow Donor Program. N Engl J Med 1993;328(9):593–602.
11. Flomenberg N, Baxter-Lowe LA, Confer D, et al. Impact of HLA class I and class II high-resolution matching on outcomes of unrelated donor bone marrow trans-plantation: HLA-C mismatching is associated with a strong adverse effect on transplantation outcome. Blood 2004;104(7):1923–30.
12. Bray RA, Hurley CK, Kamani NR, et al. National marrow donor program HLA matching guidelines for unrelated adult donor hematopoietic cell transplants. Biol Blood Marrow Transplant 2008;14(Suppl 9):45–53.
13. Lee SJ, Klein J, Haagenson M, et al. High-resolution donor-recipient HLA match-ing contributes to the success of unrelated donor marrow transplantation. Blood 2007;110(13):4576–83.
14. Goulmy E, Schipper R, Pool J, et al. Mismatches of minor histocompatibility anti-gens between HLA-identical donors and recipients and the development of graft-versus-host disease after bone marrow transplantation. N Engl J Med 1996;334(5):281–5.
15. Bleakley M, Riddell SR. Molecules and mechanisms of the graft-versus-leukaemia effect. Nat Rev Cancer 2004;4(5):371–80.
16. Goulmy E. Human minor histocompatibility antigens: new concepts for marrow transplantation and adoptive immunotherapy. Immunol Rev 1997;157:125–40.
17. Antin JH, Ferrara JL. Cytokine dysregulation and acute graft-versus-host disease. Blood 1992;80(12):2964–8.
18. Cavet J, Middleton PG, Segall M, et al. Recipient tumor necrosis factor-alpha and interleukin-10 gene polymorphisms associate with early mortality and acute

graft-versus-host disease severity in HLA-matched sibling bone marrow transplants. Blood 1999;94(11):3941–6.

19. Lin MT, Storer B, Martin PJ, et al. Relation of an interleukin-10 promoter polymorphism to graft-versus-host disease and survival after hematopoietic-cell transplantation. N Engl J Med 2003;349(23):2201–10.

20. Dickinson AM, Charron D. Non-HLA immunogenetics in hematopoietic stem cell transplantation. Curr Opin Immunol 2005;17(5):517–25.

21. Miller JS, Soignier Y, Panoskaltsis-Mortari A, et al. Successful adoptive transfer and in vivo expansion of human haploidentical NK cells in patients with cancer. Blood 2005;105(8):3051–7.

22. Miller JS, Cooley S, Parham P, et al. Missing KIR-ligands is associated with less relapse and increased graft versus host disease (GVHD) following unrelated donor allogeneic HCT. Blood 2007;109(11):5058–61.

23. Velardi A, Ruggeri L, Alessandro, et al. NK cells: a lesson from mismatched hematopoietic transplantation. Trends Immunol 2002;23(9):438–44.

24. Holler E, Rogler G, Brenmoehl J, et al. Prognostic significance of NOD2/CARD15 variants in HLA-identical sibling hematopoietic stem cell transplantation: effect on long-term outcome is confirmed in 2 independent cohorts and may be modulated by the type of gastrointestinal decontamination. Blood 2006;107(10):4189–93.

25. Weisdorf D, Hakke R, Blazar B, et al. Risk factors for acute graft-versus-host disease in histocompatible donor bone marrow transplantation. Transplantation 1991;51(6):1197–203.

26. Eisner MD, August CS. Impact of donor and recipient characteristics on the development of acute and chronic graft-versus-host disease following pediatric bone marrow transplantation. Bone Marrow Transplant 1995;15(5):663–8.

27. Martin P, Bleyzac N, Souillet G, et al. Clinical and pharmacological risk factors for acute graft-versus-host disease after paediatric bone marrow transplantation from matched-sibling or unrelated donors. Bone Marrow Transplant 2003;32(9):881–7.

28. Gale RP, Bortin MM, van Bekkum DW, et al. Risk factors for acute graft-versus-host disease. Br J Haematol 1987;67(4):397–406.

29. Nash RA, Pepe MS, Storb R, et al. Acute graft-versus-host disease: analysis of risk factors after allogeneic marrow transplantation and prophylaxis with cyclosporine and methotrexate. Blood 1992;80(7):1838–45.

30. Vigorito AC, Azevedo WM, Marques JF, et al. A randomised, prospective comparison of allogeneic bone marrow and peripheral blood progenitor cell transplantation in the treatment of haematological malignancies. Bone Marrow Transplant 1998;22(12):1145–51.

31. Cutler C, Giri S, Jeyapalan S, et al. Acute and chronic graft-versus-host disease after allogeneic peripheral-blood stem-cell and bone marrow transplantation: a meta-analysis. J Clin Oncol 2001;19(16):3685–91.

32. Eapen M, Rubinstein P, Zhang MJ, et al. Outcomes of transplantation of unrelated donor umbilical cord blood and bone marrow in children with acute leukaemia: a comparison study. Lancet 2007;369(9577):1947–54.

33. Kurtzberg J, Laughlin M, Graham ML, et al. Placental blood as a source of hematopoietic stem cells for transplantation into unrelated recipients. N Engl J Med 1996;335(3):157–66.

34. Gluckman E, Rocha V, Boyer-Chammard A, et al. Outcome of cord-blood transplantation from related and unrelated donors. Eurocord Transplant Group and

the European Blood and Marrow Transplantation Group. N Engl J Med 1997; 337(6):373–81.

35. Laughlin MJ, Barker J, Bambach B, et al. Hematopoietic engraftment and survival in adult recipients of umbilical-cord blood from unrelated donors. N Engl J Med 2001;344(24):1815–22.

36. Wagner JE, Barker JN, DeFor TE, et al. Transplantation of unrelated donor umbilical cord blood in 102 patients with malignant and nonmalignant diseases: influence of CD34 cell dose and HLA disparity on treatment-related mortality and survival. Blood 2002;100(5):1611–8.

37. Rocha V, Labopin M, Sanz G, et al. Transplants of umbilical-cord blood or bone marrow from unrelated donors in adults with acute leukemia. N Engl J Med 2004;351(22):2276–85.

38. Grewal SS, Barker JN, Davies SM, et al. Unrelated donor hematopoietic cell transplantation: marrow or umbilical cord blood? Blood 2003;101(11): 4233–44.

39. Barker JN, Weisdorf DJ, DeFor TE, et al. Transplantation of 2 partially HLA-matched umbilical cord blood units to enhance engraftment in adults with hematologic malignancy. Blood 2005;105(3):1343–7.

40. Macmillan ML, Weisdorf DJ, Brunstein CG, et al. Acute graft-versus-host disease after unrelated donor umbilical cord blood transplantation: analysis of risk factors. Blood 2009;113(11):2410–5.

41. Storb R, Deeg HJ, Whitehead J, et al. Methotrexate and cyclosporine compared with cyclosporine alone for prophylaxis of acute graft versus host disease after marrow transplantation for leukemia. N Engl J Med 1986;314(12):729–35.

42. Hiraoka A, Ohashi Y, Okamoto S, et al. Phase III study comparing tacrolimus (FK506) with cyclosporine for graft-versus-host disease prophylaxis after allogeneic bone marrow transplantation. Bone Marrow Transplant 2001;28(2): 181–5.

43. Horowitz MM, Przepiorka D, Bartels P, et al. Tacrolimus vs. cyclosporine immunosuppression: results in advanced-stage disease compared with historical controls treated exclusively with cyclosporine. Biol Blood Marrow Transplant 1999;5(3):180–6.

44. Ratanatharathorn V, Nash RA, Przepiorka D, et al. Phase III study comparing methotrexate and tacrolimus (prograf, FK506) with methotrexate and cyclosporine for graft-versus-host disease prophylaxis after HLA-identical sibling bone marrow transplantation. Blood 1998;92(7):2303–14.

45. Ram R, Gafter-Gvili A, Yeshurun M, et al. Prophylaxis regimens for GVHD: systematic review and meta-analysis. Bone Marrow Transplant 2009;43(8): 643–53.

46. Nash RA, Antin JH, Karanes C, et al. Phase III study comparing methotrexate and tacrolimus with methotrexate and cyclosporine for prophylaxis of acute graft-versus-host disease after marrow transplantation from unrelated donors. Blood 2000;96(6):2062–8.

47. van Hooff JP, Squifflet JP, Wlodarczyk Z, et al. A prospective randomized multi-center study of tacrolimus in combination with sirolimus in renal-transplant recipients. Transplantation 2003;75(12):1934–9.

48. Kirken RA, Wang YL. Molecular actions of sirolimus: sirolimus and mTor. Transplant Proc 2003;35(Suppl 3):227S–30S.

49. Cutler C, Li S, Ho VT, et al. Extended follow-up of methotrexate-free immunosuppression using sirolimus and tacrolimus in related and unrelated donor peripheral blood stem cell transplantation. Blood 2007;109(7):3108–14.

50. Bolwell B, Sobecks R, Pohlman B, et al. A prospective randomized trial comparing cyclosporine and short course methotrexate with cyclosporine and mycophenolate mofetil for GVHD prophylaxis in myeloablative allogeneic bone marrow transplantation. Bone Marrow Transplant 2004;34(7):621–5.

51. Bornhauser M, Schuler U, Porksen G, et al. Mycophenolate mofetil and cyclosporine as graft-versus-host disease prophylaxis after allogeneic blood stem cell transplantation. Transplantation 1999;67(4):499–504.

52. Kasper C, Sayer HG, Mugge LO, et al. Combined standard graft-versus-host disease (GvHD) prophylaxis with mycophenolate mofetil (MMF) in allogeneic peripheral blood stem cell transplantation from unrelated donors. Bone Marrow Transplant 2004;33(1):65–9.

53. Mohty M, de Lavallade H, Faucher C, et al. Mycophenolate mofetil and cyclosporine for graft-versus-host disease prophylaxis following reduced intensity conditioning allogeneic stem cell transplantation. Bone Marrow Transplant 2004;34(6):527–30.

54. Vogelsang GB, Arai S. Mycophenolate mofetil for the prevention and treatment of graft-versus-host disease following stem cell transplantation: preliminary findings. Bone Marrow Transplant 2001;27(12):1255–62.

55. Niederwieser D, Maris M, Shizuru JA, et al. Low-dose total body irradiation (TBI) and fludarabine followed by hematopoietic cell transplantation (HCT) from HLA-matched or mismatched unrelated donors and postgrafting immunosuppression with cyclosporine and mycophenolate mofetil (MMF) can induce durable complete chimerism and sustained remissions in patients with hematological diseases. Blood 2003;101(4):1620–9.

56. Marmont AM, Horowitz MM, Gale RP, et al. T-cell depletion of HLA-identical transplants in leukemia. Blood 1991;78(8):2120–30.

57. Martin PJ, Hansen JA, Torok-Storb B, et al. Graft failure in patients receiving T cell-depleted HLA-identical allogeneic marrow transplants. Bone Marrow Transplant 1988;3(5):445–56.

58. O'Reilly RJ. T-cell depletion and allogeneic bone marrow transplantation. Semin Hematol 1992;29(2 Suppl 1):20–6.

59. Kottaridis PD, Milligan DW, Chopra R, et al. In vivo CAMPATH-1H prevents graft-versus-host disease following nonmyeloablative stem cell transplantation. Blood 2000;96(7):2419–25.

60. Barge RMY, Starrenburg CWJ, Falkenburg JHF, et al. Long-term follow-up of myeloablative allogeneic stem cell transplantation using Campath "in the bag" as T-cell depletion: the Leiden experience. Bone Marrow Transplant 2006; 37(12):1129–34.

61. Bacigalupo A, Lamparelli T, Bruzzi P, et al. Antithymocyte globulin for graft-versus-host disease prophylaxis in transplants from unrelated donors: 2 randomized studies from Gruppo Italiano Trapianti Midollo Osseo (GITMO). Blood 2001;98(10):2942–7.

62. Reddy P, Ferrara JL. Immunobiology of acute graft-versus-host disease. Blood Rev 2003;17(4):187–94.

63. Hill GR, Ferrara JL. The primacy of the gastrointestinal tract as a target organ of acute graft-versus-host disease: rationale for the use of cytokine shields in allogeneic bone marrow transplantation. Blood 2000;95(9):2754–9.

64. Xun CQ, Thompson JS, Jennings CD, et al. Effect of total body irradiation, busulfan-cyclophosphamide, or cyclophosphamide conditioning on inflammatory cytokine release and development of acute and chronic graft-versus-host disease in H-2-incompatible transplanted SCID mice. Blood 1994;83(8):2360–7.

65. Couriel DR, Saliba RM, Giralt S, et al. Acute and chronic graft-versus-host disease after ablative and nonmyeloablative conditioning for allogeneic hematopoietic transplantation. Biol Blood Marrow Transplant 2004;10(3):178–85.
66. Choi SW, Kitko CL, Braun T, et al. Change in plasma tumor necrosis factor receptor 1 levels in the first week after myeloablative allogeneic transplantation correlates with severity and incidence of GVHD and survival. Blood 2008;112(4):1539–42.
67. Matzinger P. The danger model: a renewed sense of self. Science 2002; 296(5566):301–5.
68. Shlomchik WD, Couzens MS, Tang CB, et al. Prevention of graft versus host disease by inactivation of host antigen-presenting cells. Science 1999; 285(5426):412–5.
69. Murai M, Yoneyama H, Ezaki T, et al. Peyer's patch is the essential site in initiating murine acute and lethal graft-versus-host reaction. Nat Immunol 2003; 4(2):154–60.
70. Teshima T, Ordemann R, Reddy P, et al. Acute graft-versus-host disease does not require alloantigen expression on host epithelium. Nat Med 2002;8(6): 575–81.
71. Reddy P, Maeda Y, Liu C, et al. A crucial role for antigen-presenting cells and alloantigen expression in graft-versus-leukemia responses. Nat Med 2005; 11(11):1244–9.
72. Duffner UA, Maeda Y, Cooke KR, et al. Host dendritic cells alone are sufficient to initiate acute graft-versus-host disease. J Immunol 2004;172(12):7393–8.
73. Maeda Y, Reddy P, Lowler KP, et al. Critical role of host gammadelta T cells in experimental acute graft-versus-host disease. Blood 2005;106(2):749–55.
74. Merad M, Hoffmann P, Ranheim E, et al. Depletion of host Langerhans cells before transplantation of donor alloreactive T cells prevents skin graft-versus-host disease. Nat Med 2004;10(5):510–7.
75. Nachbaur D, Kircher B, Eisendle K, et al. Phenotype, function and chimaerism of monocyte-derived blood dendritic cells after allogeneic haematopoietic stem cell transplantation. Br J Haematol 2003;123(1):119–26.
76. Sorror ML, Maris MB, Storer B, et al. Comparing morbidity and mortality of HLA-matched unrelated donor hematopoietic cell transplantation after nonmyeloablative and myeloablative conditioning: influence of pretransplantation comorbidities. Blood 2004;104(4):961–8.
77. Korngold R, Sprent J. Negative selection of T cells causing lethal graft-versus-host disease across minor histocompatibility barriers. Role of the H-2 complex. J Exp Med 1980;151(5):1114–24.
78. Beilhack A, Schulz S, Baker J, et al. In vivo analyses of early events in acute graft-versus-host disease reveal sequential infiltration of T-cell subsets. Blood 2005;106(3):1113–22.
79. Kloosterman TC, Tielemans MJ, Martens AC, et al. Quantitative studies on graft-versus-leukemia after allogeneic bone marrow transplantation in rat models for acute myelocytic and lymphocytic leukemia. Bone Marrow Transplant 1994; 14(1):15–22.
80. Weijtens M, van Spronsen A, Hagenbeek A, et al. Reduced graft-versus-host disease-inducing capacity of T cells after activation, culturing, and magnetic cell sorting selection in an allogeneic bone marrow transplantation model in rats. Hum Gene Ther 2002;13(2):187–98.
81. Cobbold S, Martin G, Waldmann H. Monoclonal antibodies for the prevention of graft-versus-host disease and marrow graft rejection. The depletion of T cell subsets in vitro and in vivo. Transplantation 1986;42(3):239–47.

82. Sun Y, Tawara I, Toubai T, et al. Pathophysiology of acute graft-versus-host disease: recent advances. Transl Res 2007;150(4):197–214.
83. Greenwald RJ, Freeman GJ, Sharpe AH. The B7 family revisited. Annu Rev Immunol 2005;23:515–48.
84. Cohen JL, Boyer O. The role of CD4+CD25hi regulatory T cells in the physiopathogeny of graft-versus-host disease. Curr Opin Immunol 2006;18(5): 580–5.
85. Stanzani M, Martins SL, Saliba RM, et al. CD25 expression on donor CD4+ or CD8+ T cells is associated with an increased risk of graft-versus-host disease following HLA-identical stem cell transplantation in humans. Blood 2003;103(3):1140–6.
86. Rezvani K, Mielke S, Ahmadzadeh M, et al. High donor FOXP3-positive regulatory T-cell (Treg) content is associated with a low risk of GVHD following HLA-matched allogeneic SCT. Blood 2006;108(4):1291–7.
87. Ziegler SF. FOXP3: of mice and men. Annu Rev Immunol 2006;24:209–26.
88. Ferrara JL, Reddy P. Pathophysiology of graft-versus-host disease. Semin Hematol 2006;43(1):3–10.
89. Rolink AG, Gleichmann E. Allosuppressor- and allohelper-T cells in acute and chronic graft-vs.-host (GVH) disease. III. Different Lyt subsets of donor T cells induce different pathological syndromes. J Exp Med 1983;158(2):546–58.
90. Zeiser R, Nguyen VH, Beilhack A, et al. Inhibition of CD4+CD25+ regulatory T-cell function by calcineurin-dependent interleukin-2 production. Blood 2006; 108(1):390–9.
91. Krenger W, Falzarano G, Delmonte J Jr, et al. Interferon-gamma suppresses T-cell proliferation to mitogen via the nitric oxide pathway during experimental acute graft-versus-host disease. Blood 1996;88(3):1113–21.
92. Yang YG, Dey BR, Sergio JJ, et al. Donor-derived interferon gamma is required for inhibition of acute graft-versus-host disease by interleukin 12. J Clin Invest 1998;102(12):2126–35.
93. Moore KW, de Waal Malefyt R, Coffman RL, et al. Interleukin-10 and the interleukin-10 receptor. Annu Rev Immunol 2001;19:683–765.
94. Lin MT, Storer B, Martin PJ, et al. Genetic variation in the IL-10 pathway modulates severity of acute graft-versus-host disease following hematopoietic cell transplantation: synergism between IL-10 genotype of patient and IL-10 receptor beta genotype of donor. Blood 2005;106(12):3995–4001.
95. Holler E, Roncarolo MG, Hintermeier-Knabe R, et al. Prognostic significance of increased IL-10 production in patients prior to allogeneic bone marrow transplantation. Bone Marrow Transplant 2000;25(3):237–41.
96. Banovic T, MacDonald KP, Morris ES, et al. TGF-beta in allogeneic stem cell transplantation: friend or foe? Blood 2005;106(6):2206–14.
97. van den Brink MR, Burakoff SJ. Cytolytic pathways in haematopoietic stem-cell transplantation. Nat Rev Immunol 2002;2(4):273–81.
98. Wysocki CA, Panoskaltsis-Mortari A, Blazar BR, et al. Leukocyte migration and graft-versus-host disease. Blood 2005;105(11):4191–9.
99. Pribila JT, Quale AC, Mueller KL, et al. Integrins and T cell-mediated immunity. Annu Rev Immunol 2004;22:157–80.
100. Iwasaki A, Medzhitov R. Toll-like receptor control of the adaptive immune responses. Nat Immunol 2004;5(10):987–95.
101. Abhyankar S, Gilliland DG, Ferrara JL. Interleukin-1 is a critical effector molecule during cytokine dysregulation in graft versus host disease to minor histocompatibility antigens. Transplantation 1993;56(6):1518–23.

102. Tanaka J, Imamura M, Kasai M, et al. Cytokine gene expression in peripheral blood mononuclear cells during graft-versus-host disease after allogeneic bone marrow transplantation. Br J Haematol 1993;85(3):558–65.

103. Antin JH, Weisdorf D, Neuberg D, et al. Interleukin-1 blockade does not prevent acute graft-versus-host disease: results of a randomized, double-blind, placebo-controlled trial of interleukin-1 receptor antagonist in allogeneic bone marrow transplantation. Blood 2002;100(10):3479–82.

104. Martin P, Schoch G, Fisher L, et al. A retrospective analysis of therapy for acute graft-versus-host disease: initial treatment. Blood 1990;76(8):1464–72.

105. Filipovich AH, Weisdorf D, Pavletic S, et al. National Institutes of Health consensus development project on criteria for clinical trials in chronic graft-versus-host disease: I. Diagnosis and staging working group report. Biol Blood Marrow Transplant 2005;11(12):945–56.

106. Przepiorka D, Weisdorf D, Martin P, et al. 1994 Consensus Conference on Acute GVHD Grading. Bone Marrow Transplant 1995;15(6):825–8.

107. Cahn JY, Klein JP, Lee SJ, et al. Prospective evaluation of 2 acute graft-versus-host (GVHD) grading systems: a joint Société Française de Greffe de Moëlle et Thérapie Cellulaire (SFGM-TC), Dana Farber Cancer Institute (DFCI), and International Bone Marrow Transplant Registry (IBMTR) prospective study. Blood 2005;106(4):1495–500.

108. Vogelsang GB, Lee L, Bensen-Kennedy DM. Pathogenesis and treatment of graft-versus-host disease after bone marrow transplant. Annu Rev Med 2003; 54:29–52.

109. Goker H, Haznedaroglu IC, Chao NJ. Acute graft-vs-host disease: pathobiology and management. Exp Hematol 2001;29(3):259–77.

110. Choi SW, Islam S, Greenson JK, et al. The use of laparoscopic liver biopsies in pediatric patients with hepatic dysfunction following allogeneic hematopoietic stem cell transplantation. Bone Marrow Transplant 2005;36(10): 891–6.

111. Snover DC, Weisdorf SA, Ramsay NK, et al. Hepatic graft versus host disease: a study of the predictive value of liver biopsy in diagnosis. Hepatology 1984; 4(1):123–30.

112. Nevo S, Enger C, Swan V, et al. Acute bleeding after allogeneic bone marrow transplantation: association with graft versus host disease and effect on survival. Transplantation 1999;67(5):681–9.

113. Snover DC, Weisdorf SA, Vercellotti GM, et al. A histopathologic study of gastric and small intestinal graft-versus-host disease following allogeneic bone marrow transplantation. Hum Pathol 1985;16(4):387–92.

114. Paczesny S, Levine JE, Braun TM, et al. Plasma biomarkers in graft-versus-host disease: a new era? Biol Blood Marrow Transplant 2008;15(Suppl 1):33–8.

115. Paczesny S, Krijanovski OI, Braun TM, et al. A biomarker panel for acute graft-versus-host disease. Blood 2009;113(2):273–8.

116. Weisdorf D, Haake R, Blazar B, et al. Treatment of moderate/severe acute graft-versus-host disease after allogeneic bone marrow transplantation: an analysis of clinical risk features and outcome. Blood 1990;75(4):1024–30.

117. MacMillan ML, Weisdorf DJ, Wagner JE, et al. Response of 443 patients to steroids as primary therapy for acute graft-versus-host disease: comparison of grading systems. Biol Blood Marrow Transplant 2002;8(7):387–94.

118. Bertz H, Afting M, Kreisel W, et al. Feasibility and response to budesonide as topical corticosteroid therapy for acute intestinal GVHD. Bone Marrow Transplant 1999;24(11):1185–9.

119. Hockenbery DM, Cruickshank S, Rodell TC, et al. A randomized, placebo-controlled trial of oral beclomethasone dipropionate as a prednisone-sparing therapy for gastrointestinal graft-versus-host disease. Blood 2007;109(10):4557–63.
120. Shapira MY, Bloom AI, Or R, et al. Intra-arterial catheter directed therapy for severe graft-versus-host disease. Br J Haematol 2002;119(3):760–4.
121. Deeg HJ. How I treat refractory acute GVHD. Blood 2007;109(10):4119–26.
122. Alousi AM, Weisdorf DJ, Logan BR, et al. Etanercept, mycophenolate, denileukin or pentostatin plus corticosteroids for acute graft vs. host disease: a randomized phase II trial from the BMT CTN. Blood 2009;114:511–7.
123. Lamioni A, Parisi F, Isacchi G, et al. The immunological effects of extracorporeal photopheresis unraveled: induction of tolerogenic dendritic cells in vitro and regulatory T cells in vivo. Transplantation 2005;79(7):846–50.
124. Gatza E, Rogers CE, Clouthier SG, et al. Extracorporeal photopheresis reverses experimental graft-versus-host disease through regulatory T cells. Blood 2008; 112(4):1515–21.
125. Greinix HT, Knobler RM, Worel N, et al. The effect of intensified extracorporeal photochemotherapy on long-term survival in patients with severe acute graft-versus-host disease. Haematologica 2006;91(3):405–8.
126. Perfetti P, Carlier P, Strada P, et al. Extracorporeal photopheresis for the treatment of steroid refractory acute GVHD. Bone Marrow Transplant 2008;42(9): 609–17.
127. Calore E, Calo A, Tridello G, et al. Extracorporeal photochemotherapy may improve outcome in children with acute GVHD. Bone Marrow Transplant 2008; 42(6):421–5.
128. Berger M, Pessolano R, Albiani R, et al. Extracorporeal photopheresis for steroid resistant graft versus host disease in pediatric patients: a pilot single institution report. J Pediatr Hematol Oncol 2007;29(10):678–87.
129. Ringden O, Uzunel M, Rasmusson I, et al. Mesenchymal stem cells for treatment of therapy-resistant graft-versus-host disease. Transplantation 2006;81(10): 1390–7.
130. Le Blanc K, Frassoni F, Ball L, et al. Mesenchymal stem cells for treatment of steroid-resistant, severe, acute graft-versus-host disease: a phase II study. Lancet 2008;371(9624):1579–86.
131. Socie G, Stone JV, Wingard JR, et al. Long-term survival and late deaths after allogeneic bone marrow transplantation. Late Effects Working Committee of the International Bone Marrow Transplant Registry. N Engl J Med 1999;341(1): 14–21.
132. Lee SJ, Vogelsang G, Flowers ME. Chronic graft-versus-host disease. Biol Blood Marrow Transplant 2003;9(4):215–33.
133. Weiden PL, Flournoy N, Sanders JE, et al. Antileukemic effect of graft-versus-host disease contributes to improved survival after allogeneic marrow transplantation. Transplant Proc 1981;13(1 Pt 1):248–51.
134. Lee SJ, Klein JP, Barrett AJ, et al. Severity of chronic graft-versus-host disease: association with treatment-related mortality and relapse. Blood 2002;100(2): 406–14.
135. Pavletic SZ, Smith LM, Bishop MR, et al. Prognostic factors of chronic graft-versus-host disease after allogeneic blood stem-cell transplantation. Am J Hematol 2005;78(4):265–74.
136. Shulman HM, Sullivan KM, Weiden PL, et al. Chronic graft-versus-host syndrome in man. A long-term clinicopathologic study of 20 Seattle patients. Am J Med 1980;69(2):204–17.

137. Couriel D, Carpenter PA, Cutler C, et al. Ancillary therapy and supportive care of chronic graft-versus-host disease: National Institutes of Health consensus development project on criteria for clinical trials in chronic Graft-versus-host disease: V. Ancillary Therapy and Supportive Care Working Group Report. Biol Blood Marrow Transplant 2006;12(4):375–96.

138. Martin PJ, Storer BE, Rowley SD, et al. Evaluation of mycophenolate mofetil for initial treatment of chronic graft-versus-host disease. Blood 2009;113(21): 5074–82.

139. Zaja F, Bacigalupo A, Patriarca F, et al. Treatment of refractory chronic GVHD with rituximab: a GITMO study. Bone Marrow Transplant 2007;40(3): 273–7.

140. Cutler C, Miklos D, Kim HT, et al. Rituximab for steroid-refractory chronic graft-versus-host disease. Blood 2006;108(2):756–62.

141. Svegliati S, Olivieri A, Campelli N, et al. Stimulatory autoantibodies to PDGF receptor in patients with extensive chronic graft-versus-host disease. Blood 2007;110(1):237–41.

142. Olivieri A, Locatelli F, Zecca M, et al. Imatinib for refractory chronic graft-versus-host disease with fibrotic features. Blood 2009;114(3):709–18.

143. Rizzo JD, Curtis RE, Socie G, et al. Solid cancers after allogeneic hematopoietic cell transplantation. Blood 2009;113(5):1175–83.

144. Kumar A, Teuber SS, Gershwin ME. Intravenous immunoglobulin: striving for appropriate use. Int Arch Allergy Immunol 2006;140(3):185–98.

145. Kulkarni S, Powles R, Treleaven J, et al. Chronic graft versus host disease is associated with long-term risk for pneumococcal infections in recipients of bone marrow transplants. Blood 2000;95(12):3683–6.

146. Ho VT, Zahrieh D, Hockenberg D, et al. Safety and efficacy of denileukin diftitox in patients with steroid-refractory acute graft versus host disease after allogeneic hemutopoietic stem cell transplantation. Blood 2004;104(4): 1224–6.

147. Shaughnessy PJ, Bachier C, Grimley M, et al. Denileukin diftitox for the treatment of steroid-resistant acute graft-versus-host disease. Biol Blood Marrow Transplant 2005;11(3):188–93.

148. Levine JE, Paczesny S, Mineishi S, et al. Etanercept plus methylprednisolone as initial therapy for acute graft-versus-host disease. Blood 2008;111(4): 2470–5.

149. Bolanos-Meade J, Jacobsohn DA, Margolis J, et al. Pentostatin in steroid-refractory acute graft-versus-host disease. J Clin Oncol 2005;23(12):2661–8.

150. Basara N, Kiehl MG, Blau W, et al. Mycophenolate Mofetil in the treatment of acute and chronic GVHD in hematopoietic stem cell transplant patients: four years of experience. Transplant Proc 2001;33(3):2121–3.

151. Krejci M, Doubek M, Buchler T, et al. Mycophenolate mofetil for the treatment of acute and chronic steroid-refractory graft-versus-host disease. Ann Hematol 2005;84(10):681–5.

152. Takami A, Mochizuki K, Okumura H, et al. Mycophenolate mofetil is effective and well tolerated in the treatment of refractory acute and chronic graft-versus-host disease. Int J Hematol 2006;83(1):80–5.

153. Benito AI, Furlong T, Martin PJ, et al. Sirolimus (rapamycin) for the treatment of steroid-refractory acute graft-versus-host disease. Transplantation 2001;72(12): 1924–9.

154. von Bonin M, Stolzel F, Goedecke A, et al. Treatment of refractory acute GVHD with third-party MSC expanded in platelet lysate-containing medium. Bone Marrow Transplant 2009;43(3):245–51.

155. Shapira MY, Resnick IB, Bitan M, et al. Rapid response to alefacept given to patients with steroid resistant or steroid dependent acute graft-versus-host disease: a preliminary report. Bone Marrow Transplant 2005;36(12):1097–101.

Reduced Intensity Transplantation for Primary Immunodeficiency Disorders

Paul Veys, MBBS, FRCP, FRCPath, FRCPCH[a,b,*]

KEYWORDS

- Reduced intensity • Hematopoietic cell transplantation
- Primary immunodeficiency

It is more than 40 years since the first successful hematopoietic cell transplants (HCT) were reported in children with primary immunodeficiency disorders (PID).[1,2] Many advances have been made since that time such that most children with PID can now be cured from their otherwise lethal disorders through well-matched HCT procedures. Preexisting morbidity and infection remain the principal adverse factors for poor outcomes with HCT. To improve current results 3 aspects need to be considered: (1) earlier diagnosis; (2) well-tolerated pretransplant conditioning regimens; and (3) promotion of immune reconstitution.[3] This article addresses modifications in the conditioning regimen that might lead to further improvement in HCT outcomes.

Many children with PID have significant comorbidities at the time of HCT, and conventional myeloablative preparation may be associated with significant treatment-related toxicity. In the past decade reduced intensity transplantation (RIT) has become a well-established approach in adult patients with malignant disease, extending curative HCT to older individuals and patients with comorbidities otherwise ineligible for myeloablative procedures (reviewed in Refs.[4–6]). Because pediatric patients generally tolerate more intensive transplant approaches, myeloablative regimens are still preferred in childhood malignancies; this reluctance is compounded further by the fact that most RIT regimens use peripheral blood stem cells (PBSC) and pediatric centers have preferred bone marrow (BM) and cord blood (CB) because

[a] Department of BMT, Level 4 Westlink, Great Ormond Street Hospital for Children NHS Trust, Great Ormond Street, London, WC1N 3JH, UK
[b] Stem Cell Transplantation, Molecular Immunology Unit, University College London Institute of Child Health, 30 Guilford Street, London WC1N 1EH, UK
* Department of BMT, Level 4 Westlink, Great Ormond Street Hospital for Children NHS Trust, Great Ormond Street, London, WC1N 3JH, UK.
E-mail address: veysp@gosh.nhs.uk

Immunol Allergy Clin N Am 30 (2010) 103–124
doi:10.1016/j.iac.2009.11.003   immunology.theclinics.com
0889-8561/10/$ – see front matter © 2010 Elsevier Inc. All rights reserved.

of a lack of a survival advantage with PBSC in pediatric recipients[7] and reluctance to collect PBSC from minor donors.[8] Nevertheless, a study of the role of RIT in pediatric cancer has recently been completed under the auspices of the Pediatric Blood and Marrow Transplant Consortium of North America.[9] The study reports favorable outcomes with RIT approaches in pediatric patients with malignant disease who were ineligible for myeloablative HCT, as long as their disease was in clinical remission (CR) at the time of HCT. These survivors are likely to have the additional benefit of reduced long-term sequelae, including possible preservation of fertility and normal growth patterns.

RIT might be a more attractive option for children with nonmalignant disease as there is no requirement for high-dose chemotherapy to eradicate malignancy; graft failure, may be a concern in certain groups[10] as many patients with nonmalignant disorders have not received prior chemotherapy, however varying degrees of immunodeficiency should make rejection less of an obstacle in children with PID. RIT has been used successfully for many years in patients with marrow aplasia, in whom myeloablation is not required.

MECHANISM OF RIT

Conventional HCT prevents rejection by the use of supralethal chemotherapy to remove host-versus-graft (HVG) reactions, create marrow space and eradicate malignancy, often achieving full donor chimerism in the early months post HCT. RIT prevents rejection by the use of pre- ± post-HCT immunosuppression to achieve tolerance and a graft-versus-marrow (GVM) reaction to create space and eradicate malignancy. In this setting a stable mixed chimerism (MC) is often achieved, which may be converted to full donor chimerism, if required, by tailing immunosuppression or donor lymphocyte infusions (DLI). Unlike in malignant disease, stable MC in the diseased cell lineage is usually sufficient to cure genetic disease.

Two general approaches have been used to develop RIT regimens.[11,12] Terminology may be confusing, but so-called reduced intensity conditioning (RIC) protocols (**Fig. 1**) have been developed by replacing myeloablative agents with more immunosuppressive and less myelosuppressive properties.[13,14] Nevertheless, such protocols still contain agents capable of ablating stem cells, for example, busulfan or melphalan, but at a reduced dose compared with conventional HCT. In contrast regimens with minimal toxicity or minimal intensity conditioning (MIC) (see **Fig. 1**) are truly nonmyeloablative and contain only immunosuppressive agents. These latter regimens, developed in animal models, initially used irradiation to induce a degree of immunosuppression pre transplant, followed by posttransplant immunosuppression given to control residual host and newly infused donor, alloreactive T cells.[15] By definition MIC procedures have been associated with less toxicity than RIC HCT; however, as MIC relies solely on a GVM reaction to make marrow space, there is a suggestion that MIC HCT may be associated with an increased incidence of graft-versus-host disease (GVHD), particularly chronic GVHD (cGVHD), especially in the unrelated donor setting.

A truly nonmyeloablative/MIC regimen should not eradicate host hematopoiesis and should allow prompt autologous hematopoietic recovery without a transplant, but be sufficient to enable at least partial donor engraftment to occur post HCT.[16] In this setting initial chimerism is often mixed. In contrast, RIC regimens require HCT for prompt hematologic recovery and if the graft is rejected, prolonged aplasia may occur. Initial chimerism following RIC HCT is frequently 100% donor, but may decline thereafter in the absence of GVM, as autologous hematopoiesis recovers.

A hierarchy of conditioning intensity

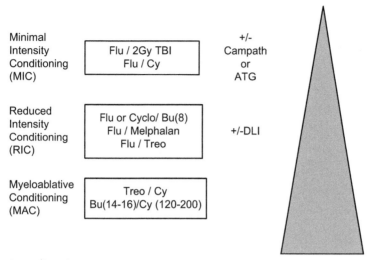

Fig. 1. A hierarchy of commonly used MIC, RIC, and MAC regimens in PID patients; Gy, gray; Flu, fludarabine; cyclo, cyclophosphamide; BU8, busulfan 8 mg/kg; BU14–16, busulfan 14–16 mg/kg; CY120–200, cyclophosphamide 120–200 mg/kg. (*From* Satwani P, Cooper N, Rao K, et al. Reduced intensity conditioning and allogeneic stem cell transplantation in childhood malignant and nonmalignant diseases. Bone Marrow Transplant 2008;41(2):174; with permission.)

RIT PROTOCOLS FOR PID

Studies reporting the use of RIT and including 5 or more patients with PID are shown in **Table 1**. Most reduced and minimal intensity protocols are based around the purine analog fludarabine, which has profound immunosuppressive and antitumor properties (see **Fig. 1**). RIC protocols combine fludarabine with a marrow ablative agent (melphalan, busulfan, or treosulfan), and MIC protocols combine fludarabine with non-marrow ablative low-dose radiation or cyclophosphamide.

RIC PROTOCOLS FOR PID
Fludarabine/Melphalan

The combination of fludarabine, melphalan, and antithymocyte globulin (ATG) (FMA) was first reported by the London group in 8 patients with severe combined immunodeficiencies (SCID) and non-SCID immunodeficiencies (see **Table 2** for definitions); despite significant comorbidities before HCT, 7 of 8 were surviving with donor cell engraftment 8 to 17 months after transplant.[17] The same group recently updated their series, reporting 113 patients with PID who had undergone RIT between 1998 and 2006.[12] Most patients (93 of 113) received a RIC regimen consisting of alemtuzumab 1 mg/kg (Campath 1H), fludarabine 150 mg/m^2, and melphalan 140 mg/m^2 (FMC), and 20 patients received MIC HCT. Donor source was mainly matched unrelated (MUD) (n = 42) and mismatched unrelated donors (mMUD) (n = 29). Eighteen patients had severe organ toxicity before transplant, including previous ventilation (n = 12), significant liver or renal impairment (n = 8), or total parental nutrition-dependent

Table 1
RIC and MIC HCT for primary immune deficiencies

Refs.	Immunodeficiency	N	Donor	Type	Conditioning	Stable Donor Chimerism	Rejection/Low-level Chimerism Requiring Further Procedure	GVHD	Survival (%)
12a	Various	113	MUD, mMUD, MRD, UCB	RIC (93) MIC (20)	Flu150 mg/m², Mel 140 mg/m², Camp or ATG (93) Flu120 mg/m², Cy40 mg/kg/anti-CD45, Camp (13)	81%	12%	2/113 died of GVHD	82
17	Various	8	MUD, MRD	RIC	Flu 120–150 mg/m², Mel 140 mg/m², ATG	86%	14%	1/8 limited cVHD	88
18b	Various	33	MUD, mMUD	RIC	Flu150 mg/m², Mel 140 mg /m², Camp or ATG	81%	19%	3/33 > grade II aGVHD, 1/33 ext cGVHD	94
19	Various	14	MUD, MRD	MIC	Flu 90 mg/m², TBI 200 cGy (10)	79% CD3 57% CD33	4/14 received second SCT/DLI/ stem cell boost	11/14 > grade II aGVHD, 8/14 ext cVHD	62
20	LAD	8	MUD, mMUD, MRD, UCB	RIC	Flu150 mg/m², Mel 140 mg/m², Camp (5) Flu150 mg/m², Treo 42 mg/m², Camp or ATG (3)	88%	1/8 MNC 30%, 0% myeloid, ? second SCT	3/8 > grade II aGVHD	100
21	SCID, WAS, HLH	5	UCB	MIC	Flu 150–180 mg/m², Cy 30–120 mg/kg ± VP16 900 mg/m², ATG	50%	2/2 HLH rejected	1/6 > grade II aGVHD	60
23	Various	6	MRD, MUD, UCB	RIC	Flu 180 mg/m², Bu (IV) 6.4 mg/kg, ATG	100%		No significant acute or ext cGVHD	67
24c	HLH	25	MUD, mMUD, UCB, Haplo MUD, MRD	RIC	Flu150 mg/m², Mel 140 mg /m², Camp (19) Flu, Mel, Camp	100%	2/25 required DLI	NA	84
	HLH/XLP	10		RIC		100%	4/10 required DLI	3/4 > grade II aGVHD post DLI	100

Ref	Disease	n	Donor		Conditioning	Chimerism	Complications	GVHD	%
25	HLH	12	mMUD, MUD, MRD Haplo	RIC	Flu150 mg/m², Mel 140 mg/m², Camp (9) Flu 150 mg/m², Mel 125 mg/m², Bu 8 mg/kg, ATG (3)	100% CD3 92% myeloid		4/12 > grade II aGVHD, 1/9 ext cGVHD	75
26	WAS	11	MUD, mMUD	RIC	Flu150 mg/m², Mel 140 mg/m², Camp (6) Treosulfan, Flu, Camp (5)	2/6 0% myeloid 1/5 0% myeloid	Splenectomy ×2	2/11 > grade II aGVHD, significant cGVHD	100
27	WAS, CGD, SCID, congenital neutropenia	6	MRD, MUD, UCB	RIC	Flu 160 mg/m², Bu ×16 doses targeted to steady-state concentration 600 ng/mL, ATG	100%	2/6 low-level myeloid	None	83
28	Various	16	MUD, mMUD, MSD, UCB	MIC	Flu 150 Cy 1200 mg/m², anti-CD45 MAbs ×2, Camp	88%	2 rejections, 1 second SCT, 3/14 no donor myeloid	6/16 > grade II aGVHD evolving to 2/16 ext cGVHD	81
29	Various	17	MSD, MUD, mMUD, UCB	RIC	Flu 150 mg/m², Treo 42 mg/m², Camp (14) or ATG (2)	88%	<50% donor in 2, ? second SCT required	2/17 > grade II aGVHD, 3/17 ext cGVHD	94
11	CGD	10	MSD	MIC	Flu 125 mg/m², Cy 120 mg/kg, ATG	80%	2 graft failures, all patients planned to receive DLIs	3/8 > grade II aGVHD, 1 evolving to ext cGVHD	70
31		6	MRD, MUD, mMUD	RIC	Flu 160 mg/m², Bu ×16 doses targeted to steady state concentration 600 ng/ml ATG (3) or Camp (3)	33%	1/6 required DLI for low level donor chimerism	1/6 grade II aGVHD evolving to ext cGVHD	100

Abbreviations: Bu, busulfan; Camp, Campath (alemtuzumab); Cy, cyclophosphamide; ext, extensive; Flu, fludarabine; Haplo, haploidentical related donor; Mel, melphalan.

[a] Includes patients from Refs. [17,18,20,24–26,29]
[b] Includes patients from Refs. [17,25,26,30]
[c] Includes patients from Cooper N, Rao K, Gilmour K, et al. Stem cell transplantation with reduced intensity conditioning for haemophagocytic lymphohistiocytosis. Blood 2006;107(3):1233–6.

Table 2
Classification of PID

■ SCID		☐ WASP Deficiency
Functional	Genetic	☐ C40 ligand deficiency (hyper-IGM)
T− B− NK−	ADA deficiency (AR)	
	Reticular dysgenesis (X-linked or AR)	☐ XLP (Purtilo syndrome)
T− B− NK+	RAG deficiency (AR)	
	SCID with Artemis (AR)	☐ Hemophagocytic syndromes
T− B+ NK−	γ deficiency (X-linked)	Immunodeficiency with partial albinism
	Jak 3 kinase deficiency (AR)	Familial HLH
T− B+NK+	IL7 Rα deficiency	Griscelli disease (partial albinism)
Unspecified		Chediak-Higashi syndrome
Other		
☐ Non-SCID		☐ Phagocytic cell disorders
☐ T-cell immunodeficiency		
CD4 lymphopenia		Schwachman syndrome
Zap 70 kinase deficiency		Granule deficiency
MHC class II deficiency		LAD
PNP deficiency		X-linked CGD
Omenn syndrome		Kostmann disease
Severe DiGeorge complex (22q 11del)		AR-CGD
CID with skeletal dysplasia		IFN-γ receptor deficiency
Cartilage hair hypoplasia		☐ Autoimmune lymphoproliferative syndrome (homozygotes) (FAS deficiency)
Other		

Abbreviations: ■, SCID; ☐, non-SCID; ADA, adenosine deaminase deficiency; AR CGD, chronic granulomatous disease; CID, combined immunodeficiency disease; IFN, interferon; MHC, major histocompatibility complex; PNP, purine nucleoside phosphorylase; RAG, recombinase activating gene; WASP, Wiskott-Aldrich syndrome protein.

enteropathy (n = 8). Five patients had DNA repair defects. At a median follow-up of 2.9 years (range 2 months–8 years) the overall survival (OS) for these patients was 82% (93 of 113) and 91 of 133 (81%) had stable donor engraftment. Fourteen patients (12%) had or were likely to require additional procedures, including second stem cell transplantation (SCT), marrow infusion, additional CD34$^+$ cells or gene therapy. The survival curve for each disease is shown in **Fig. 2**. Survival of more than 80% was observed in children receiving HCT for SCID, T-cell immune deficiency, X-linked lymphoproliferative disease (LPD), hemophagocytic lymphohistiocytosis (HLH), and Wiskott-Aldrich syndrome (WAS). As shown in **Fig. 3**, there was no significant difference in survival for patients transplanted from single-antigen mismatched donors compared with 10 of 10 HLA-matched donors, highlighting the possibility that RIC may allow HCT from less than ideal donors. Causes of death were as follows: multiorgan failure (n = 5); infection (n = 4); pneumonitis (n = 4); GVHD (n = 2); and recurrent disease, venoocclusive disease (VOD), transplant-related microangiopathy, and pulmonary hypertension (n = 1 each).

There are no prospective randomized studies comparing RIC HCT with conventional HCT in PID; however, the London group retrospectively compared their results in children with PID transplanted from unrelated donors using FMC-RIC HCT versus

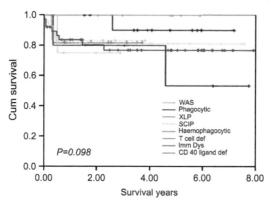

Fig. 2. OS of pediatric patients undergoing RIC SCT for PID/HLH stratified by disease. Phago-cytic, neutrophil phagocytic defect; T-cell def, isolated T-cell immunodeficiencies; Imm Dys, immunodysregulatory disorders; CD40 ligand def, CD40 ligand deficiency. (*From* Satwani P, Cooper N, Rao K, et al. Reduced intensity conditioning and allogeneic stem cell transplan-tation in childhood malignant and nonmalignant diseases. Bone Marrow Transplant 2008;41(2):176; with permission.)

myeloablative conditioning (MAC) HCT from an earlier time cohort, and showed a decreased overall mortality (2 of 33 RIC compared with 4 of 19 MAC, $P<.01$).[18] There was no difference in the incidence of acute GVHD (aGVHD), and immune reconstitu-tion with RIC was similar to that seen after conventional intensity conditioning with similar kinetics of CD19, CD3, and CD4 recovery (**Fig. 4**). There was an increase in viral infections/reactivations in the RIC cohort (29% for RIC compared with 21% following MAC, $P = .02$). Viral infections in those receiving RIC HCT included cytomegalovirus (CMV) (n = 3), adenovirus (n = 5), and Epstein-Barr virus (EBV) (n = 10). There was also an increased rate of MC compared with MAC HCT (45% MC, of which 13% had low-level donor chimerism for RIC versus 36% MC and 0% low-level donor

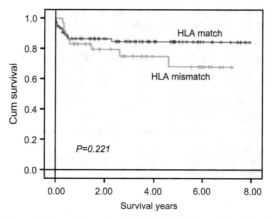

Fig. 3. OS in pediatric patients undergoing RIC HCT for PID stratified by HLA-matched versus HLA-mismatched donor. There was no significant difference in survival for HLA-matched compared with HLA-mismatched donors ($P = .2$). (*From* Satwani P, Cooper N, Rao K, et al. Reduced intensity conditioning and allogeneic stem cell transplantation in childhood malig-nant and nonmalignant diseases. Bone Marrow Transplant 2008;41(2):176; with permission.)

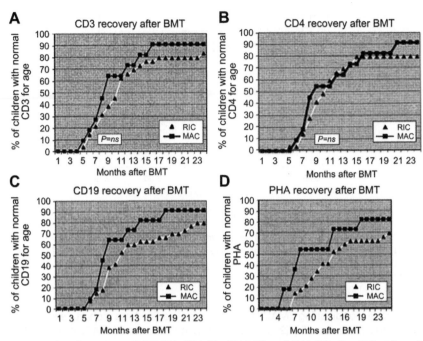

Fig. 4. Kinetics of recovery of CD3 (*A*), CD4 (*B*), CD19 (*C*) and PHA (*D*) after RIC and myeloablative transplantation (MAC) in children with primary immunodeficiencies. There was no statistical difference in speed of immune reconstitution between the 2 groups. (*From* Rao K, Amrolia P J, Jones A, et al. Improved survival after unrelated donor bone marrow transplant in children with primary immunodeficiency using a reduced intensity conditioning regimen. Blood 2005;105:884; with permission.)

chimerism for MAC); however, in general, MC after RIC appeared to stabilize or improve with withdrawal of immunosuppression, and there were low rates of recurrent disease (2 of 23 patients). OS was improved in the RIC group, mainly through improved survival in patients with non-SCID immunodeficiency (**Fig. 5**).

To assess the potential effects of the different time cohorts in this study the outcome of a larger cohort of PID patients undergoing RIC HCT from the London group was compared with that of PID patients undergoing largely MAC HCT and reported from European centers in the SCETIDE database. In this comparison (**Fig. 6**), the improvement in RIC HCT seems to be largely confined to children with T-cell deficiencies (as defined in **Table 2**).

Some of the outcomes associated with FMC/A-RIC HCT in PID have been studied further. Higher levels of viral reactivation[32] seem to relate particularly to EBV. The incidence of EBV viremia and LPD was studied in a consecutive cohort of 128 pediatric patients undergoing HCT with RIC (n = 65) or MAC (n = 68).[33] Following MAC, 6 of 68 (8%) developed viremia; all remained asymptomatic. EBV viremia (23 of 65 patients = 35%, *P*<.001) and LPD (10 of 65 = 15%, *P*<.001) were significantly more frequent following RIC. Of the 23 RIC patients who developed viremia, 8 remained asymptomatic, 5 had symptomatic viremia (fever ± rash), and 10 patients developed LPD, 2 of whom died. An absolute lymphocyte count of less than 0.3×10^9/L at the time of onset of viremia was strongly predictive of development of LPD (*P*<.05) in this group. The incidence of viremia was significantly higher in patients receiving selective T-cell

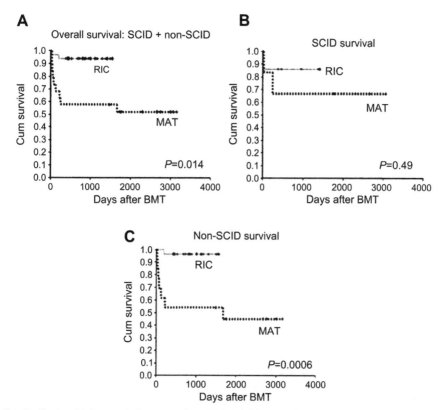

Fig. 5. Kaplan-Meier analysis comparing OS in children with primary immunodeficiencies receiving RIC or conventional conditioning (MAC or MAT) SCT. (*A*) OS in all patients was significantly better in patients who received RIC (94% OS) compared with MAC (53% OS). When divided into disease type, the improved survival following RIC was particularly marked in patients with non-SCID (who had a 54% death rate following MAC compared with a 30% death rate following MAC for SCID). (*B*) OS following either RIC or MAC in patients with SCID. (*C*) OS following RIC or MAC in patients with non-SCID. (*Reproduced from* Satwani P, Cooper N, Rao K, et al. Reduced intensity conditioning and allogeneic stem cell transplantation in childhood malignant and nonmalignant diseases. Bone Marrow Transplant 2008;41(2):176; with permission.)

depletion with ATG (15 of 43, 35%) than Campath (12 of 73, 16.4%, $P<.05$). PID and aGVHD were associated with EBV viremia in univariate analysis, but were not independent risk factors. The increased incidence of EBV viremia was believed to reflect the profound immunosuppression following RIC HCT, together with the incomplete ablation of recipient-derived B cells.[33] In contrast with this finding, the combination of FMC-RIC HCT, preemptive rituximab, and EBV-specific cytotoxic T lymphocytes was successful in curing all 8 patients with EBV-driven LPD complicating PID and immunodysregulatory syndromes,[34] suggesting that close monitoring of EBV by polymerase chain reaction and preemptive therapy mainly with rituximab can overcome complications associated with EBV viremia following RIC HCT. In adult patients a high incidence of CMV reactivation has been described following FMC-RIC HCT.[35]

Long-term chimerism (median follow-up 4.6 years, range 6 months–10.6 years) has been examined in 118 children with PID receiving FMC-RIC HCT in London (K Rao, personal communication, 2009). After prolonged follow-up donor chimerism was

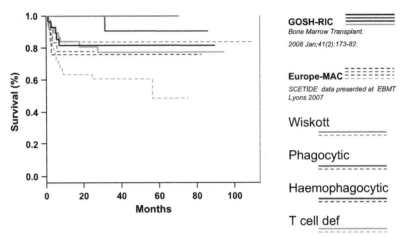

Fig. 6. Improvement in outcome of stem cell transplantation for T cell immune deficiency. GOSH-RIC, Great Ormond Street Hospital RIC HCT; Europe MAC, myeloablative HCT performed in European centers; Def, deficiency.

low (<50%) in 24 of 118 (20%) patients, 5 patients have required a second MAC HCT, 1 required a CD34+ cell top-up, 2 patients were given DLI, and 1 patient with WAS underwent a splenectomy. Twenty-one of these 24 patients are currently alive and well with stable engraftment. Two patients have died, 1 following second HCT and 1 from progressive disease, and 1 patient has continuing poor immune reconstitution. Almost all patients developing low-level donor chimerism received BM rather than peripheral blood progenitor cells (PBPC) as stem cell source and MSD and MFD had more low MC than MUDs and mMUDs (30% and 28% vs 18% and 11%). These findings have confirmed those of an earlier published study.[32] Low (<10%) donor chimerism was almost entirely limited to the myeloid series. Cyclosporin withdrawal seemed to have a positive effect on lymphoid chimerism but not on myeloid engraftment. Lymphoid chimerism changed little after the first year but myeloid chimerism did decrease further after 1 year in a few patients. Consequently, 5 years following RIC HCT for PID just less than 10% of patients have required a second procedure. This finding is probably not different from the situation following MAC HCT.

Shenoy and colleagues[36] used FMC-RIC HCT in 16 patients with nonmalignant disorders, including 2 PID patients, but gave Campath 1H 33 or 48 mg total dose early pre-HCT from day −21 to day −19. The study included sibling BM (n = 5), sibling PBSC (n = 5), unrelated BM (n = 3), and unrelated CB (n = 3). All 14 evaluable patients had complete or high-level (>50%) donor chimerism in all lineages, suggesting that lower doses or administration of Campath 1H away from the graft may increase donor chimerism in the HLA-matched setting. Further studies are under way to examine whether Campath levels taken on or around day zero may predict graft outcome in these patients (ie, high levels predicting for slow immune reconstitution and viral infections, and low levels for GVHD and complete donor chimerism). These results may better help to define the optimal method of delivering Campath in the RIT setting (Ref.[12] and S Adams, personal communication, 2007).

In addition to T cells, natural killer (NK) cells may be important in determining chimeric status post RIT. NK cells react with their target cell HLA class I molecules through killer immunoglobulinlike receptors (KIRs), which exist in inhibitory and activating forms. Following RIT, in which donor and recipient hematopoiesis may coexist, the balance of activating/inhibitory KIR activity between donor/recipient NK cells and their targets may determine chimeric status (eg, recipients with overall lower inhibitory KIR scores have more active antidonor immune effector cells, leading to reduced donor chimerism).[37]

The benefit from FMC-RIC HCT was most evident in children more than 1 year of age. For SCID patients less than 1 year of age, treatment-related mortality (TRM) remained high even with RIC HCT (28% in the London series).[28] Occasionally, very young patients seem to develop a fatal melphalan shock syndrome with massive capillary leak within hours of receiving melphalan (K Rao, personal observation, 2008), although the mechanism of this is not understood. An alternative RIC or MIC protocol (see later discussion) might be preferable for this group of patients.

Fludarabine/Busulfan

Jacobsohn and colleagues[23] reported the outcome of RIC HCT in patients with nonmalignant disorders, using fludarabine, busulfan, and ATG (FBA) modeled after Slavin and colleagues.[13] Six children with PID underwent MSD PBSC (n = 2), MUD PBSC (n = 2), and unrelated CB (n = 2) HCT. Patients received fludarabine 180 mg/m², and intravenous (IV) busulfan 6.4 mg/kg in 8 doses on days −5 to −4 or pharmacokinetic monitoring to achieve an area under the curve (AUC) of 3800 to 4200 μmol/min with single daily dosing of busulfan on days −5 and −4. Two patients with X-linked hyper-IgM were phenotypically cured, off intravenous immunoglobulin, and with reversal of cholangiopathy. One had full donor and one 30% donor chimerism. One patient with X-linked lymphoproliferative disorder (XLP) was also alive and well, with 98% donor chimerism. One patient with SCID was too early to evaluate and 2 patients (1 with chronic granulomatous disease [CGD] and 1 with Omenn disease) died within 100 days of HCT. There was little aGVHD or cGVHD in evaluable patients.

Horn and colleagues[27] also reported the use of FBA in 6 children with PID. The conditioning regimen consisted of IV busulfan from day −9 to −6, to a total of 16 doses targeting continuous steady-state concentration of 600 ng/mL. Fludarabine (40 mg/m²/d) was given from day −5 to −2 (total dose 160 mg/m²) and rabbit ATG (thymoglobulin) 0.5 mg/kg/d on day −4 and 2.5 mg/kg on days −3 to −1 (total dose 8 mg/kg). Donors were MUD BM (3), matched related BM (2), and umbilical cord blood (UCB). Three patients achieved more than 95% donor chimerism and 3 were mixed chimeras. One patient with WAS died of CMV pneumonitis; the others are alive and disease-free. There were 13 other non-PID patients included in the study; overall MC was more common with BM as a stem cell source and graft rejection was more common in patients receiving mMUDs. Four patients experienced graft failure; all 4 patients underwent second HCT and 3 of 4 are alive and disease-free, illustrating how second HCT after failed first RIC HCT is well tolerated and frequently successful.

Further work may establish an AUC for IV busulfan that is tailored to disease, donor type and stem cell source, to achieve lineage-specific donor engraftment with the minimum amount of acute and long-term toxicity. A similar protocol was used in 5 further children with PID.[31] All are alive and disease free, one patient with chronic granulomatous disease required DLI for low level donor chimerism, the others have stable or increasing mixed chimerism not requiring intervention expect one patient with complete donor chimerism who experienced siginificant acute and chronic GVHD. Interestingly in this study investigators prolonged immunosuppression for mixed chimerism rather than tailing it as the usual course of action, this did not appear to increase graft rejection though it might have reduced donor chimerism in this group.

Fludarabin/Treosulfan

Another approach to RIT in PID has been to replace busulfan with treosulfan. Treosulfan (L-threitol-1,4-bis-methanesulphonate) is the prodrug of L-epoxybutane, an alkylating agent with myeloablative and immunosuppressive properties.[29] Recent reports in adult patients have suggested that regimens containing treosulfan provide effective HCT conditioning with reduced risk of VOD, when compared with busulfan.[38–40] In addition, there is no need for prophylactic anticonvulsant treatment and unlike busulfan, it is not necessary to measure drug levels. Phase 1 studies have suggested stable linear pharmacokinetics of treosulfan up to the clinically effective dose of 42 g/m^2.[40] Eighteen patients with PID with a mean age more than 1 year underwent HCT, with various donors and stem cell sources, using treosulfan 14 g/m^2 × 3 days + fludarabine 30 mg/m^2 × 5 days with Campath 1H (FTC) (n = 14) or ATG (FTA) (n = 2).[29] One patient received cyclophosphamide 50 mg/m^2 × 4 days and ATG. Although the latter is considered modified conditioning it should probably be classified as MAC rather than RIC (see **Fig. 1**). The median time to neutrophil recovery was 12 days (9–33 days), platelet recovery 20 days (10–145 days). Thirteen patients achieved 100% donor chimerism, which remained stable in 10 patients. Three achieved stable MC: 90% to 99% donor (n = 2); 30% donor in peripheral blood, 80% donor T cells (n = 1), which was sufficient to cure the underlying disease. Two patients achieved low-level donor chimerism (<50%) and are being considered for second HCT. Twelve patients experienced no GVHD, grade I aGVHD (n = 2), grade II aGVHD (n = 1), or grade III aGVHD (n = 1) progressing to cGVHD of skin and gut. Two patients developed de novo cGVHD (limited in one and extensive skin and gut in the second). Toxicity was tolerable, particularly given such a young group of patients, and this treatment may be preferable to FMC-RIC in this cohort; toxicity included dermatologic grade II (n = 4); gut grade III (n = 9); T-cell sequestration (n = 3); pulmonary hypertension (n = 1), and right external iliac thrombosis (n = 1). Seventeen of 18 were alive at follow-up of 429 days (156–722 days). One patient had died on day 249 with cGVHD, rotavirus, and HLH.

MIC
Fludarabine/Low-Dose Total Body Irradiation

The Seattle group investigated an MIC regimen in 14 patients (12 children and 2 adults) with PID and coexisting infections, organ toxicity, or other factors precluding conventional HCT.[19] Most patients received 200 cGy total body irradiation (TBI) plus fludarabine (30 mg/m^2/d; × 3 days −4 to −2) as conditioning and all patients received HLA-matched grafts with intensive postgraft immunosuppression with cyclosporin A (CsA)/mycophenolate mophetil (MMF). No serotherapy was given. Thirteen patients established mixed (n = 5) or full (n = 8) donor chimerism and 1 rejected the graft. OS at 3 years was 62%, with a TRM of 23%. Eight of 10 evaluable patients had correction of immune deficiency with stable donor engraftment. However, there was a high rate of GVHD with 11 of 14 developing significant aGVHD (mostly grade II), and extensive cGVHD in 8 patients, reflecting the use of peripheral blood as the stem cell source and the absence of serotherapy. This approach was associated with a lower incidence of viral infections/reactivations, notably EBV, than RIC regimens using serotherapy; however, the high incidence of cGVHD is a significant obstacle to broader use of this regimen in children with nonmalignant disorders.

Fludarabine/Cyclophosphamide/Monoclonal Antibodies

The London group has explored an MIC protocol combining fludarabine (30 mg/m^2 × 5 day −8 to −4) and low-dose cyclophosphamide (300 mg/m^2 × 4 on day −7 to −4) with 2 rat anti-C45 monoclonal antibodies (MAbs) YTH 24.5/YTH 54.12 for additional myelosuppression, and serotherapy with Campath 1H either 0.6 mg/kg or 0.3 mg/kg with unrelated donor or MSD, respectively.[28] Patients were at particularly high risk from HCT-related toxicity even with RIC protocols because of severe preexisting organ toxicity, age less than 1 year, or the presence of DNA/telomere repair disorders. In total 16 patients underwent MIC HCT from MSD (5), MUD (9), and mMUD (2). Conditioning was well tolerated, with only 2 cases of grade 3 and no grade 4 toxicity. Six of 16 patients (38%) developed significant aGVHD (3 grade II skin and 3 grade III skin/gut). Five of 16 patients (31%) developed cGVHD (limited in 3 and extensive in 2), which has resolved in all cases. The incidence of GVHD was reduced when BM was used as stem cell source (2 of 10 BM recipients compared with 4 of 4 evaluable PBSC recipients developed aGVHD > grade II). Similarly the incidence of cGVHD was lower in recipients of BM (2 of 10) compared with PBSC (3 of 4). At a median of 9.5 days (range 1–15 days), 16 of 16 patients had a neutrophil count more than 0.5×10^9/L. One patient failed to engraft and had autologous recovery, and 1 patient who received a mismatched CB engrafted with stable MC after an extended period. Donor chimerism was 100% in 3 of 4 PBSC recipients, with 1 PBSC recipient rejecting the graft. Three of 10 BM recipients achieved 100% donor chimerism, 3 achieved stable high-level MC in mononuclear and granulocyte lineages, and 3 achieved donor T-cell chimerism without sustained myeloid chimerism. One achieved very-low-level donor chimerism and required a second SCT. At a median of 37 months post HCT 13 of 16 patients in this high-risk cohort were alive and cured from their underlying disease. In terms of OS, SCID patients more than 1 year of age seemed to gain particular benefit from this MIC HCT protocol (**Fig. 7**).

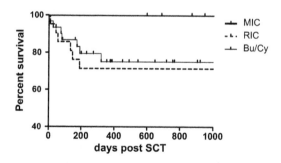

Fig. 7. Comparison of disease-free survival (DFS) of SCID patients more than 1 year of age transplanted using anti-CD45 MAb-based MIC, fludarabine/melphalan-based RIC and busulfan/cyclophosphamide conditioning. Kaplan-Meier curves showing DFS (days) of SCID patients aged more than 1 year conditioned with (1) CD45 MAb-based MIC regimen (n = 8, DFS 100%) (2) fludarabine/melphalan-based RIC regimen (n = 21, DFS 71.4%) and (3) busulfan/cyclophosphamide-based conditioning (n = 31, DFS 77.4%). The cohort conditioned with CD45-based MIC was transplanted between 2003 and 2007 (donor source 63% MUD, 25% MMUD, 13% MSD, 37% B[neg] phenotype), the cohort conditioned with fludarabine/melphalan was transplanted between 1999 and 2003 (donor source 81% MUD, 19% MMUD, 57% B[neg] phenotype) and the cohort transplanted with busulfan/cyclophosphamide was transplanted between 2003 and 2005 (donor source 57% MUD, 30% MSD, 13% MFD, 46% B[neg] phenotype).

STEM CELL SOURCE

In children with leukemia undergoing MAC HCT from MSDs, hematopoietic recovery was faster after PBSC transplantation compared with BM, risks of grade 2 to 4 acute GVHD were similar, but chronic GVHD risk was higher after PBSC transplantation. In contrast to reports in adults, TRM, treatment failure, and mortality were higher after PBSC transplantation; risks of relapse were similar.[7] The use of PBSC as opposed to BM in RIT seems to be associated with improved donor chimerism in recipients with PID,[19,28,32] but at the cost of increased rates of GVHD; in this setting OS seems to be similar between the 2 groups. The balance of HVG and GVH/GVM reflects the complex interactions of stem cell source with disease type, conditioning regimen, serotherapy, graft content (CD34+, CD3+, NK) and GVHD prophylaxis, and is more finely balanced in RIT than MAC HCT. The optimal combinations for PID remain to be determined, but even then there is likely to remain a risk of rejection with RIT and early warning of future graft rejection as suggested by recipient chimerism status in NK-cells on day +28[41] or increasing MC greater than 30% host cells[31] might enable timely intervention by withdrawl of immune suppression or DLI.

There has been increasing interest in the use of UCB in PID but using largely mye-loablative preparations (reviewed in Ref.[42]); UCB has the advantage of immediate access and a lower rate of GVHD, making it a particularly attractive stem cell source for children with PID. Several articles have been published in recent years combining RIT with UCB in more than 300 adults with malignant disease,[43] but there is considerably less experience in the use of RIT with UCB in children and even less with PID. Bradley and colleagues[21] described the outcome of 21 children, median age 9 years (range 0.33–20 years) with malignant (n = 14) and nonmalignant conditions (n = 7) transplanted using heterogeneous RIC/MIC regimens. Five patients (HLH [n = 2], SCID [n = 2], and WAS) received 4–6 of 6 HLA-matched unrelated UCB following MIC conditioning with fludarabine, cyclophosphamide, and ATG. The HLH patients received additional VP16, but both rejected; 1 underwent a successful second MAC HCT. Two of the 3 remaining patients died of viral pneumonitis and GVHD-related complications. The London group transplanted 3 patients with PID using a MIC protocol as described by Barker and colleagues.[22] Only 1 of 3 survived, 1 dying from disseminated cryptosporidiosis and the other from idiopathic pneumonitis (K Rao, personal communication, 2005). Based on only a few patients, therefore, the combination of MIC and unrelated UCB does not initially seem to offer any survival advantage to PID patients. Two centers in the UK (London and Newcastle) have performed 13 RIC UCB HCTs using fludarabine + melphalan or fludarabine + treosulfan. The outcome looks more promising, with 11 of 13 patients surviving with donor engraftment (K Rao and A Gennery, personal communication, 2009).

RIT IN SPECIFIC PID DISEASES

PID covers a large group of heterogeneous diseases (see **Table 2**). Outcomes following conventional HCT vary according to donor type and disease type: B− SCID has a poorer prognosis than B+ SCID; amongst non-SCID immunodeficiencies, T-cell deficiencies do worse than WAS, hemophagocytic diseases, and phagocytic disorders.[44] The possible advantage of RIC HCT in T-cell deficiencies has been discussed earlier, and it is likely that other specific PID types may respond differently to RIT.

HLH

Patients with HLH often have significant pretransplant comorbidities and require intensive cardiorespiratory support pre-HCT. This toxicity results in a high TRM with conventional MAC, mostly from noninfectious pulmonary toxicity and VOD. In the HLH94 study, which advocated MAC HCT, the TRM was 30%,[45] with a 3-year OS of 71% following an MFD transplant, 70% for MUD, 54% for mMUD, and 50% for those with a haploidentical donor. The use of RIT has therefore been examined closely in HLH.[24,25] Twenty-five consecutive patients with primary HLH underwent RIT in London using MUD (n = 8), mMUD (n = 11), MFD (n = 2), and haploidentical (n = 4) donors. Patients were conditioned with fludarabine 30 mg/m^2 × 5 (days −7 to −3) and melphalan 140 mg/m^2 (day −2) in patients receiving MFD/UD transplants or 125 mg/m^2 (day −1) in patients receiving haploidentical grafts. Patients receiving MFD/UD transplants received serotherapy with Campath 1H 0.2 mg/kg × 5 (days −8 to −4) and those receiving haploidentical transplants received ATG 5 mg/kg (days −5 to −1) together with busulfan 4 mg/kg (days −9 to −8) for additional myelo-suppression. One patient received a modified RIC haploidentical protocol with addition of thiotepa (10 mg/kg) to fludarabine/melphalan and OKT3 instead of ATG (P Bader, personal communication, 2007). Two patients underwent MIC HCT: one who was ventilated at the time of transplant received fludarabine 30 mg/m^2 × 3 (days −4 to −2) and 2 Gy TBI in a single fraction; and the other patient received fludarabine 120 mg/m^2, CY 30 mg/m^2, Campath 1H and 2 anti-CD45 MAbs as described earlier. Grafts were T-replete marrow (MFD/MUD) or PBSC (mMUD) and G-CSF mobilized CD34 selected or CD3/CD19 depleted PBSC (CliniMACs) for the haploidentical donors. Following RIT, 21 of 25 (84%) children are alive and in CR at a median of 36 months from transplant (range 2–105 months) with Lansky scores of 90% to 100%. There were 4 TRMs from CMV pneumonitis (n = 1), multifactorial pneumonitis following T-cell sequestration, and CMV disease on the background of previous pulmonary HLH (n = 1), parainfluenza pneumonitis (n = 1) and hepatic rupture post-transjugular liver biopsy (n = 1). No patient developed VOD. Nine patients had CMV reactivation and 9 reactivated EBV. All patients engrafted with a median of 14 days to neutrophil engraftment and a median of 16 days to an unsupported platelet count greater than 20 × 10^9/L. All patients had 100% donor cells at engraftment. Six of the 21 survivors subsequently developed MC. No patient rejected the grafts or relapsed. After this study 2 patients with progressive mixed donor chimerism received escalating DLI from their MUDs. One converted from zero to full donor myeloid chimerism, but remains 50% donor in the CD3+ fraction, and the other remained unchanged with 75% donor myeloid chimerism and 0% donor myeloid (K Rao, personal communication, 2009). Seventeen patients were alive at follow-up after more than 14 months. All of those assessed had achieved normal T-cell levels and function, as assessed by phytohemagglutinin (PHA) stimulation index, at a median of 7.5 months from SCT. One patient with X-linked lymphoproliferative syndrome had decreased NK T (CD3$^+$CD56$^+$) cells before transplant, which increased to normal levels post transplant (2.9 × 10^5/L −2.08 × 10^6/L) and remains in remission. The OS data compare favorably with historical data, particularly for patients receiving mismatched HCT (**Table 3**). In the RIT group, 7 of 8 patients (87%) transplanted from an MUD and 9 of 11 (82%) transplanted from an HLA-mismatched donor survive in CR, compared with corresponding figures of 70% and 54% in the HLH 94 study.

Further published studies of RIC HCT in patients with HLH are limited; however, an abstract presented at the Histiocyte Society Meeting 2007[46] describes 100% survival in 10 children with HLH (n = 7) or X-linked lymphoproliferative syndrome (n = 3) treated with an FMC-RIC HCT. Six patients developed MC, with 4 receiving repeated T-cell infusions. All 10 are alive and well and remain in remission at a median of 10 months. Three further patients with HLH have now undergone UD (n = 2) or RIC (n = 1) haploidentical HCT with addition of thiotepa (10 mg/kg) to fludarabine/

Table 3
Comparison of MAC versus RIC HCT for hemophagocytic lymphohistiocytosis

Donors	Historical MAC[24] (%)[a]	GOSH-RIC (%)[25]
OS	64 (86)	88 (25)
MUD	70 (33)	87 (8)
MMUD	54 (13)	82 (11)
Haploidentical	50 (16)	75 (4)
MFD	71 (24)	100 (2)

Abbreviation: GOSH, Great Ormond Street Hospital.
[a] The total number of patients in each group is described in parentheses.
Data on results with MAC are from Horne A, Janka G, Maarten Egeler R, et al. Hematopoietic stem cell transplantation in haemophagocytic lymphohistiocytosis. Br J Haematol 2005;129:622–30, whereas data on RIC are adapted from Cooper N, Rao K, Goulden N, et al. The use of reduced-intensity stem cell transplantation in haemophagocytic lymphohistiocytosis and Langerhans cell histiocytosis. Bone Marrow Transplant 2008;42(Suppl 2):S48; with permission.

melphalan and G-CSF mobilized CD3/CD19 depleted PBSC (CliniMACs) and OKT3. All 3 are alive and engrafted albeit with short follow-up (K Rao and P Bader, personal communication, 2009). Fludarabine/melphalan-based RIC HCT therefore seems to be a promising approach for children with HLH, with 34 of 38 patients surviving in initial studies. RIC HCT may be particularly suitable for children with poorly responding disease.

WAS

A recent study from the European centers examined the long-term outcome of 96 WAS patients who underwent HCT following a MAC regimen between 1979 and 2001 and who survived for at least 2 years following HCT.[47] Events included in the analysis of the 96 patients included cGVHD, autoimmunity, infections, and sequelae before or after HCT. Overall, the 7-year event-free survival was 75%, and was significantly influenced by donor group: MSD HCT, 88%; UD HCT, 71% ($P = .03$); and mMRD, 55% ($P = .003$). cGVHD-independent autoimmunity in 20% of patients was strongly associated with mixed or split (donor T-cell, host myeloid, and B-cell) chimerism status, suggesting that residual host cells can moderate autoimmune disease despite coexistence of donor cells. The overall incidence of autoimmunity was 8% in patients with full donor chimerism and 71% in patients with mixed/split chimerism ($P = .001$). This finding might have significant implications for the use of RIT in WAS, as RIT has been associated with increased rates of MC.[18] Conversely, WAS patients more than 5 years old who have accumulated more comorbidities have a poorer outcome following MAC HCT,[48] and RIT may offer some advantages in this setting. Investigators in London have explored the use of RIC HCT in WAS (updated from Ref.[46]). Between 1995 and 2007, 17 patients with WAS with a median age of 27 months underwent MSD (n = 5) or UD HCT (n = 12). MAC (busulfan/cyclophosphamide) was used in 6 patients, and RIC HCT in 11: treosulfan/fludarabine (n = 5), fludarabine/melphalan (n = 6). Amongst the 11 patients receiving RIC 10 had WAS and 1 X-linked thrombocytopenia. The mean age in this group was 70 months (15–194 months) and the mean Ochs score was 4.8. Donor source was MUD (n = 10) and mMUD (n = 1). Eight patients received BM and 3 patients PBSC. All patients survive, with a median follow-up of 4 years. Five of the 17 patients have mixed/split chimerism (details shown in **Table 3**) all following UD HCT: 1 of 2 following MAC UD HCT, and 4 of 11 (36%) following RIC UD HCT. All 4 of these patients received in vivo T-cell depletion with Campath 1H 1 mg/kg total dose day −8 to day −4. Only 1 of these patients has so far developed definite autoimmune disease (**Table 4**). Three subsequent patients underwent UD HCT with RIT with reduced Campath 1H 0.6 mg/kg total dose day −8 to day −6, and all achieved 100% donor chimerism, with only 1 patient experiencing aGVHD grade II skin. Three of four patients with MC developed aGVHD higher than grade II, as opposed to 3 of 15 with full donor chimerism (*P*<.05). Comparative incidence of mixed/split chimerism following MAC HCT in other studies is 28%[47] and 38%.[49] RIC HCT protocols may be suitable for UD HCT in WAS, particularly in older children with comorbidities; however, some GVM reaction is required to secure 100% donor chimerism in all patients.

CGD

Horwitz and colleagues[50] reported 10 patients with CGD who underwent MIC HCT comprising cyclophosphamide (120 mg/kg), fludarabine (125 mg/m^2) and ATG (160 mg/kg), followed by transplant of CD34+-selected peripheral blood mononuclear cells from MSDs. Delayed DLI was given at intervals of 30 or more days to increase the level of donor chimerism. After a median follow-up of 17 months donor myeloid chimerism in 8 of 10 patients ranged from 33% to 100%, a level that could be expected to provide normal host defense. In 2 patients graft rejection occurred. Significant aGHVD developed in 3 of 4 adult patients with engraftment, 1 of whom

Table 4
Patients with WAS who became mixed chimeras after HCT

Presentation Ochs Score	Donor	Conditioning	Donor Chimerism (%)	Autoimmune Disease
Petechiae AHA Rituximab Infections 5	MUD BM	Treosulfan 42 g/m^2 Fludarabine 150 mg/m^2 Campath 1H 1.0 mg/kg	CD3 76 CD15 0 CD19 29	No splenectomy
Petechiae Eczema Infections 4	MUD BM	Melphalan 140 mg/m^2 Fludarabine 150 mg/m^2 Campath 1H 1.0 mg/kg	CD3 100 WB <5	AHA Splenectomy
Petechiae Infections Arthritis Splenectomy 5	MUD BM	Melphalan 140 mg/m^2 Fludarabine 150 mg/m^2 Campath 1H 1.0 mg/kg	CD3 80 CD15 0 CD19 52	No
Petechiae GI bleed Cerebral bleed Splenectomy 5	mMUD PBPC	Treosulfan 42 g/m^2 Fludarabine 150 mg/m^2 Campath 1H 1.0 mg/kg	CD3 100 CD15 63	No
IC bleed GI bleed Retuximab Splenectomy 5	MUD PBSC	Busulfan 16 mg/kg Cyclophos 200 mg/kg Campath 1H 1.0 mg/kg	CD3 62 CD15 58 CD19 53	No

Abbreviations: AHA, autoimmune hemolytic anemia; cyclophos, cyclophosphamide; GI, gastrointestinal; IC, intracranial.

subsequently had extensive cGVHD. Seven patients were reported to have survived from 16 to 26 months. Two patients died of transplant-related complications, and 1 patient who rejected the graft died after a second HCT.

As a comparison RIC HCT using FBA, busulfan 8 to 10 mg/kg (adjusted with busulfan kinetics in pediatric patients), fludarabine 180 mg/m², and ATG 40 mg/kg and matched donors (MSD = 5, MUD = 3) in 8 high-risk CGD patients led to 90% to 100% donor chimerism at a median follow-up of 26 months.[51,52] This is despite the use of BM in 7 of 8 cases. Seven patients are alive and well, and all active inflammatory and infectious foci are cured. One adult patient who had received PBSC from a CMV-negative MUD died of CMV pneumonitis on day +150. Another type of RIC HCT (4 Gy of TBI, cyclophosphamide 50 mg/kg, and fludarabine 200 mg/m²) followed by 2 mismatched unrelated CB units in a single adult McLeod phenotype CGD patient with invasive aspergillosis also resulted in full donor engraftment and cure.[53] All 5 CGD patients who received FMC-RIC HCT survived, but sustained donor engraftment was achieved in only 2 of 5 (T Gungor, personal communication, 2008). RIC HCT using the FBA combination may be particularly suitable for high-risk patients with CGD.[30]

Leukocyte Adhesion Deficiency

The transplant experience for 36 children with leukocyte adhesion deficiency (LAD) undertaken at 14 centers worldwide between 1993 and 2007 was recently surveyed.[20] At a median follow-up of 62 months OS was 75%. MAC was used in 28 patients, and the remaining 8 patients received RIC (FMC = 5, FTC/A = 2) Survival after MFD and UD transplants was similar, with 11 of 14 MFD and 12 of 14 UD recipients surviving; mortality was greatest after haploidentical HCT, in which 4 of 8 children did not survive. Full donor chimerism was achieved in 17 of the survivors, mixed multilineage chimerism in 7 patients, and mononuclear cell restricted chimerism in a further 3 patients. Causes of death in the 9 patients who died included pneumonitis (n = 2), infection (n = 5), VOD (n = 3), and malignancy (n = 1); some had more than 1 contributing factor and all had received MAC HCT. Overall, the use of RIC regimens seemed to be associated with reduced toxicity, with all 8 patients surviving, although 2 patients have low-level donor chimerism, not requiring second HCT to date.

FERTILITY AND LATE EFFECTS

One major impetus for performing RIT in children is the avoidance or reduction of long-term sequelae associated with MAC HCT, including growth failure, gonadal failure, secondary malignancies, and myelodysplasia.[54] However, the true incidence of late effects following RIT in children with PID awaits well-planned and well-executed follow-up studies as the first cohorts of survivors approach adulthood. Intact fertility and uncomplicated pregnancies have been reported in dogs with canine LAD following MIC HCT.[55] There have been several reports of successful pregnancies in adults following FMC- and FBA-RIC protocols for malignant disease. One adult CGD patient fathered a child after FBA[51]; however the impact of the same drugs on the pediatric gonadal and endocrine systems may be different. The avoidance of busulfan on the developing brain might have been considered to have a beneficial effect on cognitive function and improve IQ, but conditioning type seemed to have no impact on these parameters in the PID population.[56]

SUMMARY

Studies so far indicate that RIT may have an important role in treating patients with PID. Unlike more standard approaches, such regimens can be used without severe toxicity in patients with severe pulmonary or hepatic disease. RIT also offers the advantage that long-term sequelae such as infertility or growth retardation may be avoided or reduced. Prospective randomized studies are required to define the true benefit of RIT versus MAC in any given type of PID; such studies are unlikely given the small number of patients and physician and patient/family preferences. On the present evidence the use of RIT seems to be most appropriate for those patients with significant comorbidities (eg, T-cell deficiencies) and those undergoing UD HCT. More studies are required using pharmacokinetic monitoring (eg, busulfan and Campath 1H) and varying stem cell sources to optimize GVM reactions and minimize GVHD. In certain PID patients RIT will be the first step toward establishing donor cell engraftment; second infusions of donor stem cells, DLI, or a second MAC HCT (which seems to be well tolerated) may be required in some patients with low-level donor chimerism or graft rejection.

REFERENCES

1. Gatti RA, Meuwissen HJ, Allen HD, et al. Immunological reconstitution of sex-linked lymphopenic immunological deficiency. Lancet 1968;2(7583):1366–9.
2. Bach FH, Albertini RJ, Joo P, et al. Bone-marrow transplantation in a patient with the Wiskott-Aldrich syndrome. Lancet 1968;2(7583):1364–6.
3. Filipovich A. Hematopoietic cell transplantation for correction of primary immunodeficiencies [review]. Bone Marrow Transplant 2008;42(Suppl 1):S49–52.
4. Alousi A, de Lima M. Reduced-intensity conditioning allogeneic hematopoietic stem cell transplantation. Clin Adv Hematol Oncol 2007;5:560–70.
5. Barrett AJ, Savani BN. Stem cell transplantation with reduced-intensity conditioning regimens: a review of ten years experience with new transplant concepts and new therapeutic agents. Leukemia 2006;20:1661–72.
6. Rezvani AR, Storb R. Using allogeneic stem cell/T-cell grafts to cure hematologic malignancies. Expert Opin Biol Ther 2008;8:161–79.
7. Eapen M, Horowitz MM, Klein JP, et al. Higher mortality after allogeneic peripheral-blood transplantation compared with bone marrow in children and adolescents: the Histocompatibility and Alternate Stem Cell Source Working Committee of the International Bone Marrow Transplant Registry. J Clin Oncol 2004;22:4872–80.
8. Pulsipher MA, Nagler A, Iannone R, et al. Weighing the risks of G-CSF administration, leukopheresis, and standard marrow harvest: ethical and safety considerations for normal pediatric hematopoietic cell donors. Pediatr Blood Cancer 2006;46:422–33.
9. Pulsipher MA, Boucher KM, Wall D, et al. Reduced-intensity allogeneic transplantation in pediatric patients ineligible for myeloablative therapy: results of the Pediatric Blood and Marrow Transplant Consortium Study ONC0313. Blood 2009;114(7):1429–36.
10. Iannone R, Casella JF, Fuchs EJ, et al. Results of minimally toxic nonmyeloablative transplantation in patients with sickle cell anemia and beta-thalassemia. Biol Blood Marrow Transplant 2003;9:519–28.
11. Woolfrey A, Pulsipher MA, Storb R. Nonmyeloablative hematopoietic cell transplant for treatment of immune deficiency [review]. Curr Opin Pediatr 2001;13(6):539–45.
12. Satwani P, Cooper N, Rao K, et al. Reduced intensity conditioning and allogeneic stem cell transplantation in childhood malignant and nonmalignant diseases [review]. Bone Marrow Transplant 2008;41(2):173–82.

13. Slavin S, Nagler A, Naparstek E, et al. Nonmyeloablative stem cell transplantation and cell therapy as an alternative to conventional bone marrow transplantation with lethal cytoreduction for the treatment of malignant and nonmalignant hematologic diseases. Blood 1998;91(3):756–63.

14. Champlin R, Khouri I, Shimoni A, et al. Harnessing graft-versus-malignancy: non-myeloablative preparative regimens for allogeneic haematopoietic transplantation, an evolving strategy for adoptive immunotherapy. Br J Haematol 2000;111: 18–29.

15. Storb R, Yu C, Wagner JL, et al. Stable mixed hematopoietic chimerism in DLA-identical littermate dogs given sublethal total body irradiation before and pharmacological immunosuppression after marrow transplantation. Blood 1997; 89(8):3048–54.

16. Giralt S, Estey E, Albitar M, et al. Engraftment of allogeneic hematopoietic progenitor cells with purine analog-containing chemotherapy: harnessing graft-versus-leukemia without myeloablative therapy. Blood 1997;89:4531–6.

17. Amrolia P, Gaspar B, Hassan A, et al. Non-myeloablative stem cell transplantation for congenital immunodeficiencies. Blood 2000;96:1239–46.

18. Rao K, Amrolia PJ, Jones A, et al. Improved survival after unrelated donor bone marrow transplant in children with primary immunodeficiency using a reduced intensity conditioning regimen. Blood 2005;105:879–85.

19. Burroughs LM, Storb R, Leisenring WM, et al. Intensive post-grafting immune suppression combined with nonmyeloablative conditioning for transplantation of HLA-identical hematopoietic cell grafts: results of a pilot study for treatment of primary immunodeficiency disorders. Bone Marrow Transplant 2007;40:633–42.

20. Qasim W, Cavazzana-Calvo M, Davies EG, et al. Allogeneic hematopoietic stem-cell transplantation for leukocyte adhesion deficiency. Pediatrics 2009;123(3): 836–40.

21. Bradley MB, Satwani P, Baldinger L, et al. Reduced intensity allogeneic umbilical cord blood transplantation in children and adolescent recipients with malignant and non-malignant diseases. Bone Marrow Transplant 2007;40(7):621–31.

22. Barker JN, Weisdorf DJ, DeFor TE, et al. Rapid and complete donor chimerism in adult recipients of unrelated donor umbilical cord blood transplantation after reduced-intensity conditioning. Blood 2003;102(5):1915–9.

23. Jacobsohn DA, Duerst R, Tse W, et al. Reduced intensity haemopoietic stem-cell transplantation for treatment of non-malignant diseases in children. Lancet 2004; 364:156–62.

24. Cooper N, Rao K, Goulden N, et al. The use of reduced-intensity stem cell transplantation in haemophagocytic lymphohistiocytosis and Langerhans cell histiocytosis. Bone Marrow Transplant 2008;42(Suppl 2):S47–50.

25. Cooper N, Rao K, Gilmour K, et al. Stem cell transplantation with reduced intensity conditioning for haemophagocytic lymphohistiocytosis. Blood 2006;107(3): 1233–6.

26. Ochs HD, Filipovich AH, Veys P, et al. Wiskott-Aldrich syndrome: diagnosis, clinical and laboratory manifestations, and treatment. Biol Blood Marrow Transplant 2008;15(Suppl 1):84–90.

27. Horn B, Baxter-Lowe LA, Englert L, et al. Reduced intensity conditioning using intravenous busulfan, fludarabine and rabbit ATG for children with nonmalignant disorders and CML. Bone Marrow Transplant 2006;37(3):263–9.

28. Straathof KC, Rao K, Eyrich M, et al. Haemopoietic stem cell transplantation with antibody-based minimal intensity conditioning regimen for children with severe organ toxicity or DNA repair disorders. Lancet 2009;374:912–20.

29. Greystoke B, Bonanomi S, Carr TF, et al. Treosulfan-containing regimens achieve high rates of engraftment associated with low transplant morbidity and mortality in children with non-malignant disease and significant co-morbidities. Br J Haematol 2008;142:257–62.
30. Seger RA. Modern management of chronic granulomatous disease. Br J Haematol 2008;140(3):255–66.
31. Ozyurek E, Cowan MJ, Koerper MA, et al. Increasing mixed chimerism and the risk of graft loss in children undergoing allogeneic hematopoietic stem cell transplantation for non-malignant disorders. Bone Marrow Transplant 2008;42(2): 83–91.
32. Veys P, Rao K, Amrolia P. Stem cell transplantation for congenital immunodeficiencies using reduced-intensity conditioning. Bone Marrow Transplant 2005; 35(Suppl 1):S45–7.
33. Cohen J, Gandi M, Naik P, et al. Increased incidence of EBV-related disease following paediatric stem cell transplantation with reduced-intensity conditioning. Br J Haematol 2005;129(2):229–39.
34. Cohen JM, Sebire NJ, Harvey J, et al. Successful treatment of lymphoproliferative disease complicating primary immunodeficiency/immunodysregulatory disorders with reduced-intensity allogeneic stem cell transplantation. Blood 2007;110(6): 2209–14.
35. Chakrabarti S, Mackinnon S, Chopra R, et al. High incidence of cytomegalovirus infection after nonmyeloablative stem cell transplantation: potential role of Campath-1H in delaying immune reconstitution. Blood 2002;99(12): 4357–63.
36. Shenoy S, Grossman WJ, DiPersio J, et al. A novel reduced-intensity stem cell transplant regimen for nonmalignant disorders. Bone Marrow Transplant 2005; 35(4):345–52.
37. Sobecks RM, Ball EJ, Askar M, et al. Influence of killer immunoglobulin-like receptor/HLA ligand matching on achievement of T-cell complete donor chimerism in related donor nonmyeloablative allogeneic hematopoietic stem cell transplantation. Bone Marrow Transplant 2008;41(8):709–14.
38. Casper J, Knauf W, Blau I, et al. Treosulfan/fludarabine: a new conditioning regimen in allogeneic transplantation. Ann Hematol 2004;83(Suppl 1):S70–1.
39. Casper J, Knauf W, Kiefer T, et al. Treosulfan and fludarabine: a new toxicity-reduced conditioning regimen for allogeneic hematopoietic stem cell transplantation. Blood 2004;103:725–31.
40. Beelen DW, Trenschel R, Casper J, et al. Dose-escalated treosulphan in combination with cyclophosphamide as a new preparative regimen for allogeneic haematopoietic stem cell transplantation in patients with an increased risk for regimen-related complications. Bone Marrow Transplant 2005;35:233–41.
41. Matthes-Martin S, Lion T, Hass OA, et al. Lineage-specific chimaerism after stem cell transplantation in children following reduced intensity conditioning: potential predictive value of NK cell chimaerism for late graft rejection. Leukemia 2003;17: 1934–42.
42. Gennery AR, Cant AJ. Cord blood stem cell transplantation in primary immune deficiencies [review]. Curr Opin Allergy Clin Immunol 2007;7(6):528–34.
43. Chen YB, Spitzer TR. Current status of reduced-intensity allogeneic stem cell transplantation using alternative donors. Leukemia 2008;22(1):31–41.
44. Antoine C, Muller S, Cant A, et al. Long term survival and haematopoietic stem cell transplantation for immunodeficiencies: a survey of the European experience 1968–1999. Lancet 2003;361:553–60.

45. Horne A, Janka G, Maarten Egeler R, et al. Haematopoietic stem cell transplantation in haemophagocytic lymphohistiocytosis. Br J Haematol 2005;129: 622–30.
46. Vaughn G, Bleesing J, Jordan M, et al. Hematopoietic cell transplantation with reduced intensity conditioning (RIC HCT) for hemophagocytic lymphohistiocytosis (HLH) and X-linked lymphoproliferative syndrome [abstract]. Proceedings of the Histiocyte Society Meeting, Cambridge, September 2007. p. 20.
47. Ozsahin H, Cavazzana-Calvo M, Notarangelo LD, et al. Long-term outcome following hematopoietic stem cell transplantation in Wiskott-Aldrich syndrome: collaborative study of the European Society for Immunodeficiencies and the European Group for Blood and Marrow Transplantation. Blood 2008;111(1):439–45.
48. Filipovich AH, Stone JV, Tomany SC, et al. Impact of donor type on outcome of bone marrow transplantation for Wiskott-Aldrich syndrome: collaborative study of the International Bone Marrow Transplant Registry and the National Marrow Donor Program. Blood 2001;97(6):1598–603.
49. Pai SY, DeMartiis D, Forino C, et al. Stem cell transplantation for the Wiskott–Aldrich syndrome: a single-center experience confirms efficacy of matched unrelated donor transplantation. Bone Marrow Transplant 2006;38:671–9.
50. Horwitz ME, Barrett AJ, Brown MR, et al. Treatment of chronic granulomatous disease with nonmyeloablative conditioning and a T-cell-depleted hematopoietic allograft. N Engl J Med 2001;344(12):881–8.
51. Güngör T, Halter J, Klink A, et al. Successful low toxicity hematopoietic stem cell transplantation for high-risk adult chronic granulomatous disease patients. Transplantation 2005;79(11):1596–606.
52. Gungor T, Halter J, Stussi G, et al. Successful busulphan-based reduced intensity conditioning in high-risk paediatric and adult chronic granulomatous disease – The Swiss experience [abstract]. Bone Marrow Transplant 2009; 43(Suppl 1):S75.
53. Suzuki N, Hatakeyama N, Yamamoto M, et al. Treatment of McLeod phenotype chronic granulomatous disease with reduced-intensity conditioning and unrelated-donor umbilical cord blood transplantation. Int J Hematol 2007;85(1):70–2.
54. Satwani P, Morris E, Bradley MB, et al. Reduced intensity and non-myeloablative allogeneic stem cell transplantation in children and adolescents with malignant and non-malignant diseases [review]. Pediatr Blood Cancer 2008;50(1):1–8.
55. Burkholder TH, Colenda L, Tuschong LM, et al. Reproductive capability in dogs with canine leukocyte adhesion deficiency treated with nonmyeloablative conditioning prior to allogeneic hematopoietic stem cell transplantation. Blood 2006; 108(5):1767–9.
56. Titman P, Pink E, Skucek E, et al. Cognitive and behavioural abnormalities in children following haematopoietic stem cell transplantation for severe congenital immunodeficiencies. Blood 2008;112(9):3907–13.

Radiosensitive Severe Combined Immunodeficiency Disease

Christopher C. Dvorak, MD, Morton J. Cowan, MD*

KEYWORDS

- Severe combined immunodeficiency disease • Radiosensitive
- Hematopoietic cell transplant • Artemis • DNA ligase IV

Patients with severe combined immunodeficiency (SCID) disease have classically been divided into those with residual B cells (T−B+ phenotype) and those whose defects produce an absence of T cells and B cells (T−B− phenotype). The T−B− phenotype accounts for approximately 30% of patients with SCID and is associated with worse outcomes after hematopoietic cell transplantation (HCT) in most[1–4] but not all studies.[5] Various genetic mutations have now been linked to the T−B− phenotype, most of which result in defects in the protein machinery required for the variable (density) joining [V(D)J] recombination events that are critical for producing the diverse repertoire of the T- and B-cell immune system.

The first step in V(D)J recombination involves creation of double-stranded DNA (dsDNA) breaks and subsequent hairpin formation by an enzymatic complex produced by recombination activating gene (RAG)-1 and RAG-2 (**Fig. 1**). Defects in RAG also produce a T−B− form of SCID but without radiosensitivity.[6] However, once the dsDNA breaks are created by the RAG complex, proper repair must take place to avoid a differentiation arrest, which occurs in B cells at the transition from cytoplasmic Igμ− to Igμ+ pre-B cells and in T cells at the transition from progenitor T cells to double negative progenitor T cells.[7,8]

NONHOMOLOGOUS END JOINING

Eukaryotic cells possess 2 mechanisms by which dsDNA breaks are repaired: homologous recombination (HR) and nonhomologous end joining (NHEJ). Defects in genes that produce components of the HR pathway result in diseases, such as

---

Funding: National Institutes of Health 1U54 AI082973.

Division of Pediatric Blood and Marrow Transplantation, University of California, San Francisco, 505 Parnassus Avenue, M-659, San Francisco, CA 94143-1278, USA

* Corresponding author.

E-mail address: mcowan@peds.ucsf.edu (M.J. Cowan).

doi:10.1016/j.iac.2009.10.004
immunology.theclinics.com

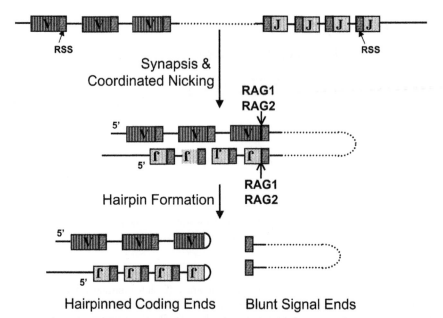

Fig. 1. V(D)J recombination: initial process and hairpin formation. RSS, recombination signal sequence. (*Adapted from* Cowan MJ. T cell negative, B cell negative, NK cell positive severe combined immunodeficiency disease. In: Basow DS, editor. UpToDate. Waltham (MA): UpTo-Date Inc; 2009; with permission. Copyright 2009 UpToDate Inc. For more information visit www.uptodate.com.)

ataxia-telangiectasia,[9] Seckel syndrome,[10] Nijmegen breakage syndrome,[11] and Fanconi anemia,[11] which are characterized by physical abnormalities with immunodeficiency and/or predisposition to cancer development.

The NHEJ pathway is especially critical in the repair of dsDNA breaks created by the RAG process during V(D)J recombination in T and B lymphocytes (**Fig. 2**). After a dsDNA break is created, the first protein that binds to the ends of the dsDNA break is a heterodimer known as Ku 80/86.[12] Ku then recruits a complex made up of 2 proteins: Artemis (also known as DNA cross-link repair enzyme 1C or DCLRE1C) and DNA-dependent protein kinase catalytic subunit (DNA-PKcs). This complex performs 2 functions via its nuclease activity. First, it opens the DNA hairpins created by the RAG complex, and second, it acts to trim the ends to variable extents, thereby contributing to functional diversity.[13] Finally, the 2 ends of DNA are ligated together, a task performed by a complex of 2 proteins: DNA ligase IV and x-ray cross-complementation group 4 (XRCC4) protein.[14,15] Another factor, known as Cernunnos-XLF, accumulates at the site of dsDNA breaks and appears to stimulate the DNA ligase IV:XRCC4 complex.[16]

AGENTS RESPONSIBLE FOR DSDNA BREAKS

Although defects in NHEJ are classically considered to produce radiosensitive forms of SCID, a wide variety of agents, other than ionizing radiation, produce dsDNA breaks via reactive oxygen species. These breaks would normally be repaired through the same NHEJ mechanism as radiation-induced damage. Cell lines from Artemis-deficient patients are moderately sensitive to mitomycin C, an alkylating agent that causes

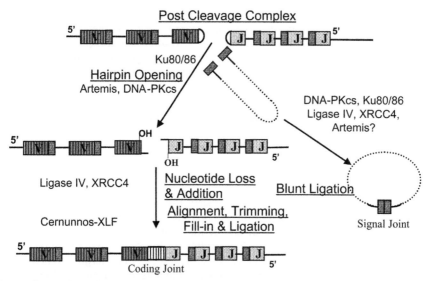

Fig. 2. The nonhomologous end-joining pathway. DNA-PKcs, DNA-dependent protein kinase catalytic subunit; XRCC4, x-ray cross-complementation group 4 (*Adapted from* Cowan MJ. T cell negative, B cell negative, NK cell positive severe combined immunodeficiency disease. In: Basow DS, editor. UpToDate. Waltham (MA): UpToDate Inc; 2009; with permission. Copyright 2009 UpToDate Inc. For more information visit www.uptodate.com.)

DNA cross-links of guanine nucleotides by attaching an alkyl group.[17] Cross-linking makes it impossible for the DNA strands to successfully uncoil and separate during the normal DNA replication process, so that affected cells are unable to divide properly. The stalled replication fork is normally repaired by the excision of the damaged area and subsequent DNA rejoining via the components of either the HR or the NHEJ pathways.

This property of alkylating agents forms the basis of their utility as anticancer chemotherapeutic agents. These chemotherapy medications were then adopted for their utility in the conditioning process to prepare a patient (including potentially a patient with SCID) to undergo an allogeneic HCT because they can target the immune system to prevent graft rejection and/or host hematopoietic cells, thereby opening niches in the bone marrow microenvironment for donor cells to attach and grow. Classic alkylating agents include those in the nitrogen mustard family (eg, cyclophosphamide and melphalan) as well as busulfan and thiotepa.[18]

Another essential component of the allogeneic HCT process is control over the alloreactive donor T cells' ability to cause graft-versus-host disease (GVHD). This has been accomplished through the use of calcineurin inhibitors, which block downstream signaling from the interleukin (IL)-2 receptor. The calcineurin inhibitor cyclosporine can produce dsDNA breaks, at least in cells deficient in DNA ligase IV.[19]

DIAGNOSTIC TESTS FOR RADIATION SENSITIVITY

Even before specific mutations in various components of the NHEJ pathway were identified, a subset of patients with T−B− SCID were known to have an increased sensitivity to ionizing radiation.[20] Initial experiments were performed by creating colony-forming unit–granulocyte-macrophage (CFU-GM) from the patient's bone marrow samples. The CFU-GM was exposed to increasing doses of irradiation (0.5–3 Gy), and the survival relative to nonirradiated cells was compared with the bone marrow from healthy age-matched controls.[20,21] The current approach to assessing radiation sensitivity involves creating primary skin fibroblasts from patients with SCID. Fibroblasts in exponential growth phase are then exposed to increasing doses of radiation (1–6 Gy) and then regrown for 10 to 14 days. Survival relative to nonirradiated cells and healthy controls is then calculated.[7,22–24] The difficulties with this approach are the acquisition of cell samples and the time it takes to generate the fibroblasts from a skin biopsy in culture (6–8 weeks) when there is a sense of urgency about doing an HCT to correct the underlying disease.

SEVERE COMBINED IMMUNODEFICIENCY SYNDROMES

Although HR can repair a wide variety of DNA damages, only NHEJ seems to be capable of repairing the hairpins formed during V(D)J recombination in T- and B-cell development. Therefore, defects in any of the proteins involved in NHEJ are not cross-repaired by HR and are thus incompatible with normal maturation of both T and B cells. However, because natural killer (NK) cells do not undergo V(D)J recombination and are thus present in normal numbers, patients with defects in NHEJ have a phenotype of T−B−NK+ SCID. The presence of normal NK cells in these patients is clinically very important because NK cells differentiate self from foreign cells based on interactions of killer immunoglobulin-like receptor (KIR) ligands with human leukocyte antigen (HLA) class I antigens. Because of this, immunocompetent NK cells in patients with radiosensitive SCID pose a significant barrier to the engraftment of HLA-mismatched donor stem cells.[25,26]

Mutations in Artemis, DNA ligase IV, DNA-PKcs, and Cernunnos-XLF have all been reported to cause SCID in humans. So far to date, human mutations in Ku or XRCC4 have not been described, although a mouse model of Ku deficiency does exist.[27] Defects in XRCC4 seem to be embryonically lethal in mice.[28]

Artemis Deficiency

The Artemis protein, in complex with DNA-PKcs, performs the crucial NHEJ function of opening the DNA hairpins created by the RAG complex and then acts to nucleolytically trim the ends to variable extents. Mutations in the Artemis gene represent the most common cause of radiosensitive SCID.

For almost 3 decades, it has been known that Native Americans from the Navajo and Apache tribes (Athabascan speakers) in the southwestern United States had an extremely high incidence of T−B−NK+ SCID (SCIDA), with an estimated 52 cases per 100,000 live births.[29] The mutation in Athabascan-speaking Native American infants with SCID was localized to chromosome 10p[30] and was eventually found to be a null mutation in the Artemis gene,[31] which had previously been identified as defective in other patients with radiosensitive T−B− SCID.[32] In addition to Athabascan-speaking Native Americans, Artemis mutations have been described in infants of European, Turkish, and Japanese descent.[32,33]

Only 1 article to date has specifically focused on the outcomes after HCT for Athabascan-related SCID.[34] However, this article was limited by the fact that it was published before the discovery of the mutation in the Artemis gene, and subsequent analysis has discovered that 2 of the patients with T−B−NK+ SCID included in this report actually had mutations in RAG-1, rather than Artemis.[24] This article still represents the largest series of Artemis-deficient patients reported, and it was the first to highlight the role of alkylating agents on growth and development of secondary teeth.

Since the discovery of the Artemis gene, several other articles have begun to specifically identify small numbers of Artemis-deficient patients who have undergone HCT **(Table 1)**.[5,7,33,35–37] Although the numbers are too small for any definitive conclusions, in general, most patients with Artemis deficiency fail to develop B cells after nonconditioned HCT and require life-long immunoglobulin replacement.[34,38] However, some patients with Artemis deficiency do survive the conditioning process and have evidence of B-cell recovery, although information regarding long-term follow-up of these patients is limited.

As to be expected, patients with Artemis deficiency seem to have an increased sensitivity to therapeutic doses of ionizing radiation. Both SCIDA patients who received total body irradiation (7 Gy) died from toxic complications.[34] Whether Artemis-deficient patients have increased late effects from nontherapeutic doses of radiation in the form of radiographs is not known. Furthermore, patients with Artemis deficiency who receive alkylator-based conditioning regimens may have growth delay and failure of permanent tooth development.[34] Among SCID patients who were alive 2 years post HCT, those with Artemis deficiency had the poorest long-term event-free survival, highest rates of infection, GVHD and/or autoimmunity, and need for nutritional support.[38]

Hypomorphic mutations in Artemis have also been described in 4 patients, resulting in a partial immunodeficiency and a predisposition to Epstein-Barr virus (EBV)-associated lymphomas.[39] Fibroblasts from these patients did show sensitivity to ionizing radiation.

DNA Ligase IV Deficiency

DNA ligase IV is a crucial enzyme in the final DNA rejoining step of NHEJ. Null mutations in DNA ligase IV are embryonically lethal in mice.[40] Hypomorphic mutations in

Table 1
Published reports of outcomes after HCT for Artemis-deficient SCID

References	Year	Number	Donor	Conditioning	Outcomes
O'Marcaigh et al[34]	2001	14	Varied	Varied	10 alive: 3 with B-cell recovery 4 dead: infection, AIHA
Noordzij et al[7]	2003	4	NR	NR	2 alive: 1 with B-cell recovery 2 dead: infection; MOF
Kobayashi et al[33]	2003	4	NR	NR	2 alive: T- & B-cell recovery 2 dead: CMV, BO
van der Burg et al[37]	2006	1	Sibling Repeat	None BU4	Alive: no B-cell recovery Alive: T- & B-cell recovery
Friedrich et al[35]	2007	2	Haplo	None	2 alive: 1 with donor B cells
Grunebaum et al[5]	2006	2 5	MUD Haplo	BU20/CY200 BU20/CY200	1 alive, 1 dead (CMV) 2 alive, 3 dead (Interstitial pneumonitis, AC)
Slatter et al[36]	2008	1 1 2	MUD Haplo Haplo	BU8/CY200 BU8/CY200 BU16/CY200	Alive: retransplanted Alive: B-cell recovery Alive: B-cell recovery

Abbreviations: AC, autoimmune cytopenia; AIHA, autoimmune hemolytic anemia; BO, bronchiolitis obliterans; BU, busulfan (# is mg/kg); CMV, cytomegalovirus; CY200, cyclophosphamide (200 mg/kg); Haplo, haploidentical donor; MOF, multiorgan failure; MUD, match unrelated donor; NR, not reported.

DNA ligase IV were first described in 4 patients as part of a syndrome associated with microcephaly, unusual facial features, growth retardation, and developmental delay, resembling Seckel syndrome, but with immunodeficiency.[41] Cell lines from these patients demonstrated pronounced radiosensitivity.

Two Moroccan siblings were reported to undergo haploidentical HCT from their mother.[42] The first patient who was conditioned with busulfan, cyclophosphamide (doses not specified), and antithymocyte globulin (ATG) developed an EBV-associated posttransplant lymphoproliferative disease (PTLD) and died.[19] The second patient who was conditioned with busulfan (8 mg/kg total dose), cyclophosphamide (200 mg/kg total dose), and ATG developed severe sinusoidal obstruction syndrome (SOS) and died.[19] Two German siblings have been described with similar features.[43] The first patient died of aspergillosis during the preparative regimen for HCT. The second patient was conditioned with thiotepa (15 mg/kg total dose), fludarabine (5.72 mg/kg total dose), and ATG and underwent matched unrelated donor bone marrow transplantation (BMT).[19] She developed microangiopathic hemolytic anemia but was surviving at 8 months post HCT. The patient reportedly had full donor chimerism and improving T-cell reconstitution (B-cell reconstitution was not reported) but significant neurodevelopmental delay.

The degree of immunodeficiency seen in ligase IV syndrome is variable. A 14-year-old Japanese girl with a ligase IV mutation and clinical features consistent with the syndrome showed evidence of a combined immunodeficiency and died from an EBV-associated lymphoma.[44] A 10-year-old German girl had only low immunoglobulin levels with recurrent otitis and respiratory tract infections but developed progressive bone marrow aplasia.[45] She was conditioned with cyclophosphamide (40 mg/kg total dose), fludarabine (120 mg/m^2 total dose), and ATG and underwent a matched sibling BMT. She achieved full donor chimerism and immune reconstitution, including response to vaccinations. Because an achievement of 100% donor chimerism is not commonly seen after nonmyeloablative HCT for Artemis deficiency,[34] it is possible that the pre-HCT bone marrow hypoplasia seen in this patient caused sufficient open niches for donor hematopoietic stem cell (HSC) engraftment to occur, which has been reported in X-linked SCID.[46]

It seems that mutations in ligase IV can also produce SCID without developmental defects and syndromic features.[47] The Turkish patient in this report appeared to have a "leaky" mutation that allowed the development of low levels of circulating B cells. The V(D)J junctions in this patient demonstrated excessive nucleotide deletions, presumably caused by prolonged exposure to the exonuclease activity of the Artemis:DNA-PKcs complex during the delayed ligation process. She presented in the 2nd year of life, later than most patients with T−B−NK+ SCID, with severe respiratory infections, perineal candidiasis, chronic diarrhea, and fever. This patient was conditioned with busulfan (approximately 8 mg/kg total dose) and cyclophosphamide (approximately 160 mg/kg total dose) and underwent a matched sibling umbilical cord blood (UCB) transplant. She developed probable SOS and died.

Although only a few patients have been reported, it seems that patients with deficiency of DNA ligase IV, either in the syndromic form or as an isolated cause of T−B−NK+ SCID, have excessive toxicity and mortality after conventional myeloablative HCT with busulfan-based conditioning comparable with what has been seen in Artemis-deficient patients.[34] In vitro exposure of DNA ligase IV-deficient cell lines has not shown an increased sensitivity to busulfan or the nonalkylators fludarabine and methotrexate, at least at the concentrations used.[19] However, it seems that cyclosporine alone, but especially in combination with busulfan and fludarabine, did cause increased dsDNA breaks. A similar effect was not seen in Artemis-deficient cells.

Finally, not all mutations in DNA ligase IV seem to cause clinical immunodeficiency because some patients have been discovered only after they exhibited excessive toxicity after therapy for cancer. A 14-year-old normal-appearing Turkish boy with T-cell acute lymphoblastic leukemia (ALL) had severe toxicity following standard doses of chemotherapy and died of encephalopathy after prophylactic cranial irradiation.[48] Later, his cells were found to harbor a mutation in DNA ligase IV.[49] A 4-year-old German-Canadian boy with clinical features of DNA ligase IV syndrome but without associated immunodeficiency was also identified after presenting with T-cell ALL.[50] After routine chemotherapy, he developed prolonged neutropenia and died of presumed sepsis. These unfortunate outcomes highlight the probable heightened sensitivity of patients with mutations in DNA ligase IV to both radiation and some chemotherapeutic agents.

DNA-PKcs Deficiency

DNA-PKcs is the partner of Artemis in DNA hairpin opening complex. Defects in the DNA-PKcs gene are known to produce SCID in mice,[51] Arabian horses,[52] and Jack Russell terriers.[53] In vitro studies have demonstrated that cells that are deficient in DNA-PKcs not only are radiosensitive but also have increased dsDNA breaks after treatment with other alkylating chemotherapeutic agents, such as nitrogen mustard,[54] melphalan,[54,55] chlorambucil,[55] and doxorubicin (Adriamycin).[55] However, DNA-PKcs cells do not show increased sensitivity to the antimetabolite 5-florouracil[55] or to the topoisomerase II inhibitor etoposide,[56] neither of which are alkylators. So far, null mutations in DNA-PKcs have not been described in humans, suggesting that this protein may play a significant role in the development of cells other than lymphocytes and null mutations may be embryonically lethal.

Recently, the first human patient with a DNA-PKcs missense mutation (L3062R) was reported.[8] The mutation did not affect the kinase activity or the DNA end-binding capacity but appeared to insufficiently activate Artemis function. Not surprisingly, this Turkish patient presented with a radiosensitive form of T−B−NK+ SCID. She did not have microcephaly or other physical stigmata, although she did present with a large aphthous ulcer, reminiscent of that described in Athabascan-speaking patients with Artemis deficiency.[34,57] She underwent a nonconditioned HCT from her HLA-identical cousin and had full recovery of B-cell numbers, although the functionality of the B cells was not reported. This would be an unusual finding because B-cell recovery is not generally seen after nonconditioned transplantation for Artemis deficiency.[34]

Cernunnos-XLF Deficiency

Cernunnos-XLF is another factor that accumulates at the site of dsDNA breaks and seems to function by stimulating the DNA ligase IV:XRCC4 complex.[16] Five patients from 4 families (French, Turkish, and Italian) composed the first report of mutations in the Cernunnos-XLF gene.[58] All patients presented with severe infections and a T−B−NK+ SCID phenotype. They also demonstrated microcephaly and growth retardation, and some had bird-like facies and/or bony malformations. One patient also had bone marrow aplasia. As expected, skin fibroblasts demonstrated an increased sensitivity to ionizing radiation, which was comparable to that seen in Artemis-deficient cells. The first 2 patients died of infection, whereas the other 3 were being supported by antibiotic and immunoglobulin prophylaxis.

The first reported HCT for a patient with Cernunnos-XLF deficiency used a reduced-intensity regimen of fludarabine (120 mg/m^2 total dose), cyclophosphamide (1200 mg/m^2 total dose), and ATG with peripheral blood stem cells from a 7/8 matched unrelated donor.[59] The patient developed grade 2 skin acute GVHD and an EBV-associated PTLD requiring treatment with 16 doses of rituximab. At 2-year follow-up, the patient had 100% donor engraftment and normal T-cell numbers but was still receiving replacement immunoglobulin for low B-cell numbers, possibly as a consequence of the prolonged rituximab therapy.

Similar to what was noted earlier in 1 patient with DNA ligase IV deficiency, achievement of 100% donor chimerism is not commonly seen after a nonmyeloablative HCT for Artemis deficiency.[34] One explanation is that the pre-HCT bone marrow hypoplasia seen in this patient may have caused sufficient open niches for donor HSC engraftment to occur. An alternate explanation is that the occurrence of acute GVHD caused by alloreactive T cells mediated host HSC destruction, thereby opening niches for the donor HSC engraftment, which has been reported in adenosine deaminase–deficient SCID.[60]

OMENN SYNDROME

Omenn syndrome, an SCID phenotype associated with erythroderma, hepatosplenomegaly, lymphadenopathy, alopecia, and elevated numbers of activated T cells with a restricted T-cell receptor repertoire is classically seen in T−B− SCID patients with hypomorphic defects in the RAG genes.[61] More recently, however, it has been appreciated that a wide variety of genetic defects can contribute to the development of Omenn syndrome, including a compound heterozygous Artemis mutation with partial activity[23] and heterozygous mutations in the DNA ligase IV gene.[62]

The presence of Omenn syndrome in a patient with an underlying radiosensitive form of SCID could prove to be problematic because the activated autologous T-cell clones in addition to the normally functioning NK cells serve as a barrier to donor cell engraftment.[61] Although pharmacologic suppression of these T cells with corticosteroids and/or cyclosporine has helped to facilitate engraftment of bone marrow from HLA-identical donors, transplantation from alternative donors without myeloablative conditioning has been associated with poor overall survival.[61] Therefore, in general, patients with Omenn syndrome undergoing alternative donor HCT are given myeloablative conditioning,[61] which in a patient with underlying radiosensitivity may be associated with long-term complications.

The previously described patient with Omenn syndrome with a defect in Artemis underwent myeloablative conditioning (exact details not reported) and an HLA-haploidentical transplant from his mother, with achievement of complete donor chimerism and normal immune function; however, long-term follow-up and details regarding possible late effects of the conditioning were lacking.[23] Of note, primary skin fibroblasts from this patient had identical radiation sensitivity as those from patients with complete Artemis deficiency,[23] indicating that a partial defect in Artemis may be sufficient to produce a potentially clinically relevant degree of radiosensitivity. The patient with Omenn syndrome caused by defects in the DNA ligase IV gene received a conditioning regimen of busulfan (16 mg/kg total dose) and cyclophosphamide (200 mg/kg total dose) and had significant short-term complications after HLA-matched unrelated donor BMT but survived. She also developed numerous late effects, including microcephaly, developmental delay, and short stature[62]; however, many of these problems are similar to the manifestations in other reported patients with DNA ligase IV syndrome, irrespective of HCT.[41] Therefore, additional patients with Omenn syndrome secondary to defects in the NHEJ complex will need to be described, with careful attention to late effects, before it is clear about how these individuals respond to myeloablative conditioning.

APPROACHES TO HCT

Currently, testing of cells from SCID patients for radiosensitivity is only available on a research basis. Therefore, the authors recommend that all newly diagnosed T−B−NK+ SCID patients be evaluated for the presence of a mutation in either of the 2 RAG genes. Sequencing of the RAG genes is commercially available. In the absence of a RAG mutation, genotyping for an Artemis mutation (also commercially available) should be done and a radiosensitive form of SCID should be assumed. Until more detailed long-term analysis of sufficient numbers of radiosensitive SCID patients has been performed, the most cautious approach to HCT would involve complete avoidance of therapeutic irradiation and use of the least amount (if any) of alkylator-based chemotherapy as possible to obtain donor cell engraftment.

Donor Selection

Radiosensitive SCID patients with HLA-matched siblings should proceed directly to bone marrow transplant without the use of pretransplant conditioning. Eradication of transplacentally acquired maternally engrafted T cells before matched sibling HCT is not necessary for subsequent donor T-cell engraftment,[34,37] possibly because the maternal T cells generally have a limited T-cell receptor diversity and are functionally anergic.[63,64] However, if maternal GVHD is present, lympholytic agents may need to be used as part of the anti-GVHD therapy. Success has been reported with both ATG[34] and fludarabine,[46] neither of which would be predicted to produce dsDNA breaks and, therefore, should not have significant toxicity for a radiosensitive SCID patient.

Cyclosporine is generally administered for 4 to 6 months after matched sibling HCT for GVHD prophylaxis. Many centers also administer a second agent, such as short-course methotrexate or mycophenolate mofetil. Although concerns exist regarding the safety of using cyclosporine in patients with DNA ligase IV deficiency, it still likely needs to be used until the use of calcineurin-inhibitor-free GVHD prophylaxis regimens are better understood. An alternate possibility for patients with ligase IV deficiency would be partial ex vivo T-cell depletion; however, this approach has not yet been reported in great detail,[65] and too vigorous removal of donor T cells could adversely affect engraftment.

In the absence of an HLA-matched sibling, use of an unrelated donor (volunteer adult or UCB) versus a haploidentical donor depends on a multitude of factors, including (1) preexisting infections at the time of presentation, (2) the relative rarity of certain ethnic groups in the unrelated donor database, and (3) local expertise with ex vivo T-cell depletion techniques.[66] One advantage of T-cell–depleted haploidentical HCT, especially for patients with DNA ligase IV deficiency, is that post-HCT administration of GVHD prophylactic medications is not needed.

If the decision is made to proceed with a haploidentical donor, the presence of transplacentally acquired, maternally engrafted T cells must be ascertained, as these cells can interfere with the engraftment of stem cells from a paternal donor.[67] The presence of pre-HCT maternally engrafted cells is associated with an increased likelihood of post-HCT T-cell engraftment when a maternal donor is used, presumably because the tolerance to maternal cells by residual host immune cells indicate permissiveness to maternal donor stem cells.[68] However, in the absence of maternal engraftment, engraftment after haploidentical HCT is less successful, presumably because of the presence of major histocompatibility barriers recognized by normally functioning host NK cells. A prospective trial designed to test the hypothesis that the administration of megadoses (approximately 20×10^6 CD34+ cells/kg recipient body weight) of haploidentical donor stem cells would improve B-cell reconstitution after nonconditioned HCT was not successful in overcoming NK-mediated graft resistance and resulted in only a 43% engraftment rate in patients without preexisting maternal engraftment.[68]

Another significant problem with haploidentical HCT has been that T-cell immunologic recovery can be slow, allowing progression of underlying infections. However, the use of megadoses of donor stem cells may result in faster T-cell recovery.[68] In addition, the use of nonspecific haploidentical donor lymphocyte infusions has been shown to be safe and potentially associated with accelerated T-cell recovery and clearance of infections.[69] Furthermore, several groups are also showing success at creating pathogen-specific T cells to be used to either treat or prevent infection after haploidentical HCT.[70–72] Finally, if poor T-cell function persists after haploidentical HCT, nonconditioned stem cell boosts have also been useful for augmenting immunity,[38,73] especially if administered less than 1 year post HCT.[74]

The decision to use an unrelated donor is associated with different problems. The search process for an unrelated donor can be lengthy, especially for patients with underrepresented ethnic backgrounds. This delay might not be tolerated if the patient presents with a serious infection. The time to transplant might be shortened if UCB is used, given its increased permissiveness of HLA mismatches and more rapid acquisition time. In addition, because virtually all radiosensitive SCID patients will be very young, the limited cell doses in UCB grafts are rarely a significant issue. However, use of an unrelated donor generally requires the use of pretransplant conditioning and post-HCT pharmacologic immunosuppression for GVHD prophylaxis.

Conditioning

The use of pre-HCT conditioning is controversial, even for patients with nonradiosensitive forms of SCID,[66] given the concerns that myeloablative doses of chemotherapy can be associated with not only short-term toxicity (such as SOS) but also infertility, hormonal deficiencies and short stature, and potentially malignancy and neurocognitive delay.[75,76] These concerns are heightened in the setting of a radiosensitive SCID patient, but formal long-term analysis of sufficient numbers of such patients is lacking. Recent data suggest that cognitive and behavioral function in SCID patients post HCT is identical between those who received conditioning therapy and those who did not; however, it should be noted that no children with radiosensitive SCID were specifically documented in this report and the overall number of patients was small.[77] Similarly, although there were no cases of true secondary malignancy (excluding EBV-mediated lymphoproliferation) post HCT in 117 patients with immunodeficiency, it is unknown whether any of these patients had radiosensitive SCID.[78] A more recent cohort of 90 patients with SCID (including 12 with Artemis deficiency) surviving more than 2 years post HCT demonstrated only 1 case of secondary myelodysplasia in a patient with reticular dysgenesis.[38]

It has been reported that among patients with T−B− SCID, only those who received myeloablative conditioning with busulfan achieved normal B-cell function post HCT.[1] Similarly, another report suggests that T−B− SCID patients have improved survival if conditioning is used.[3] Presumably the use of myeloablative chemotherapy creates space for HSC engraftment in the niches of the bone marrow. These early reports are limited, however, by the lack of molecular diagnosis of patients, so that patients with nonradiosensitive RAG deficiency are lumped together with patients with Artemis deficiency.

Furthermore, the dogma that myeloablative conditioning is absolutely required for bone marrow stem cell engraftment and subsequent B-cell recovery has been challenged by rare reports of patients with T−B−NK+ SCID who develop B-cell recovery after nonablative HCT.[34,45,68,79] An interesting report of full B-cell recovery after matched sibling HCT for Artemis-deficient SCID further demonstrates the incomplete understanding of the factors involved in B-cell recovery.[37] In this report, the patient had first undergone a nonconditioned BMT from her HLA-identical brother, with T-cell recovery but no B cells. She then underwent a second BMT from the same donor with low-dose busulfan (4 mg/kg total dose), which was well tolerated. The patient subsequently developed functional B cells of donor origin with vaccine responses but without IgA production. However, her NK cells and myeloid cells remained of host origin, suggesting that only a selective B-cell precursor graft was achieved.

Currently, almost all reported unrelated donor HCTs for the treatment of SCID use some form of pre-HCT conditioning. Theoretically, a radiosensitive SCID patient undergoing HCT from a perfectly matched unrelated donor might be expected to show evidence of T-cell recovery in a fashion similar to that seen in matched sibling HCTs because the lack of HLA class I differences would minimize NK cell alloreactivity. However, to the authors' knowledge, this has not yet been reported. Although some studies indicate that full doses of busulfan (16 mg/kg or more) can be administered to patients with radiosensitive forms of SCID, the reported toxic mortality is not insignificant and the follow-up is too limited for full understanding of the possible late effects.[5,34,36] If busulfan is to be used, then pharmacokinetic targeting is highly recommended to avoid the excessive toxicity (mucositis and SOS) associated with high levels. A concentration steady state (Css) of approximately 600 ng/mL should be sufficient for donor HSC engraftment[80]; for children with radiosensitivity, an even lower Css might suffice, although data are lacking. Another option is to use a reduced-intensity regimen of melphalan (140 mg/m^2), fludarabine (150 mg/m^2), and alemtuzumab or ATG[81,82]; however, melphalan is also an alkylator, and long-term follow-up after receiving this agent is incomplete.

For a T-cell–depleted haploidentical HCT in a patient with SCID, myeloablative-type conditioning, similar to that used for unrelated donors, has been used.[2,5,83] However, there are also successful reports using either no conditioning or solely immunoablative conditioning.[2,34,65,83] For a haploidentical HCT, the major barrier to engraftment in a T−B−NK+ radiosensitive SCID patient is the presence of the immunocompetent NK cells, which differentiate self from foreign cells based on interactions of KIRs with HLA class I antigens.[25,26] With the use of megadose CD34$^+$ cell grafts, 43% of nonmaternally engrafted patients with NK+ forms of SCID show evidence of T-cell engraftment in the absence of conditioning.[68] T-cell engraftment was seen in all 8 patients who had evidence of transplacental maternal T-cell engraftment at the time of diagnosis; thus, conditioning is not needed for these patients.[68] Therefore, the authors generally recommend a nonconditioned HCT as the initial approach. If the patient does not show evidence of T-cell recovery in a timely fashion after a nonconditioned HCT, then a repeat HCT with conditioning must be considered. If conditioning is required, at first glance, fludarabine would be a good choice because it generally has less short-term toxicity than cyclophosphamide; however, unlike cyclophosphamide,[84] fludarabine does not inhibit NK cells.[85] Serotherapy, in the form of ATG or alemtuzumab, does appear to inhibit at least some populations of NK cells, and because serotherapy should cause no long-term toxicity in radiosensitive SCID patients, it should likely be part of any haploidentical conditioning regimen.[86]

FUTURE DIRECTIONS

Now that defects in 4 of the genes involved in the NHEJ pathway are known to cause SCID and that diagnostic tests of radiosensitivity have become more available, it will soon be possible to characterize each patient's genotype before HCT. This character-ization will significantly improve the management of these patients, particularly in terms of what conditioning agents (or doses) are best avoided.

The rarity of these various disorders makes the performance of prospective hypoth-esis testing in clinical trials exceedingly difficult. Clinical trials will only be possible through large multicenter collaborations. Until those become available, murine models can help in developing novel approaches to conditioning, although not all of these models truly mimic the human disease. For example, several mouse models of Artemis deficiency have been created. The first model was limited by leakiness that allowed the production of some T cells.[87] A more recent model mimics the typical human phenotype more accurately.[88] Similar mouse models exist for DNA ligase IV,[89] DNA-PKcs,[51] and Cernunnos-XLF[90] deficiencies. These models should prove invaluable for preclinical testing of new approaches to therapy for patients with radio-sensitive forms of SCID.

One priority of preclinical testing is to determine the toxicity and the ability of currently available agents to eradicate NK cells and/or open hematopoietic niches. Ideally, these would be agents that do not produce dsDNA breaks. For example, flu-darabine,[19] azathioprine,[84] and 5-florouracil[55] produce their effects through NHEJ-repair-independent mechanisms and are thus presumably relatively safe to use in patients with radiosensitive forms of SCID. However, none of these agents have signif-icant effects on inhibiting NK cells or in creating space in the bone marrow. But by extension, newer antimetabolites, such as the significantly myelosuppressive agent clofarabine, might soon have utility in creating space for donor HSCs to engraft without significant risk for long-term effects.

An alternate approach to the creation of HSC niches would be to avoid the use of classical chemotherapy-based conditioning regimens altogether. This could poten-tially be done through the administration of agents that cause HSC to leave the marrow space, such as the CXCR4-inhibitor plerixafor (AMD3100). There are preliminary data in mice that plerixafor opens niches for donor stem cells to engraft.[91] Alternately, monoclonal antibodies to antigens expressed on HSCs, such as c-kit, could be used to eliminate HSCs.[92] Finally, donor T cells might be used to target host HSCs. This has been reported to occur spontaneously in a few patients with either ADA- or IL-2Rcγ chain-deficient SCID.[46,60] In a mouse model, pretreatment of host-sensitized naive donor T cells with photochemical therapy using psoralen and ultraviolet A light prevents proliferation but preserves their cytotoxic alloreactivity to the point where GVHD is minimized but donor HSC engraftment is facilitated.[93]

Ultimately, gene therapy may prove to be a safe and effective approach to correct the immunodeficiency that is associated with these radiosensitive disorders. To date, this has been studied in animal models of Artemis deficiency.[94,95] Results indicate that both T- and B-cell reconstitution can occur, but the technique is still limited, as it requires the use of either busulfan or total body irradiation.

SUMMARY

Inherited defects are known to occur in 4 components of the NHEJ DNA repair mech-anism to produce a T−B−NK+ SCID characterized by heightened sensitivity to radi-ation and alkylating agents. These include deficiencies of Artemis, DNA ligase IV, DNA-PKcs, and Cernunnos-XLF, but only Artemis deficiency has been found in more than a small number of patients. In addition to its role in V(D)J recombination, NHEJ is involved in repair of dsDNA breaks after exposure to ionizing radiation and possibly after many forms of alkylator-based chemotherapy. Because the follow-up of patients with radiosensitive SCID that have undergone HCT is relatively limited, the exact short- and long-term toxicities of myeloablative conditioning are unclear. Any patient with T−B−NK+ SCID without a defect in RAG should be presumed to have a radiosensitive form of SCID, and confirmatory radiation sensitivity testing should be done if possible. However, the results of this testing can take a significant time to return, and HCT should not be delayed. Testing for Artemis mutations is commercially available and should be done on all suspected radiosensitive SCID patients. Once the optimal donor has been identified, patients should proceed with the minimal amount of pre-HCT conditioning needed to overcome engraftment barriers, using agents thought not to cause a significant degree of dsDNA breaks (such as ATG or alemtuzumab) whenever possible. HLA-matched sibling donors and maternal donors, when there is a transplacental maternal engraftment, do not need pre-HCT conditioning therapy, although the likelihood of B-cell reconstitution is much lower. Radiosensitive SCID patients should be observed very closely post HCT for potential late effects and, optimally, entered into collaborative group registries or trials to capture important data regarding HCT for these rare patients. More research needs to be done in order to discover novel nontoxic approaches to HCT that might benefit not only those with radiosensitive SCID but someday potentially all patients.

REFERENCES

1. Haddad E, Landais P, Friedrich W, et al. Long-term immune reconstitution and outcome after HLA-nonidentical T-cell-depleted bone marrow transplantation for severe combined immunodeficiency: a European retrospective study of 116 patients. Blood 1998;91(10):3646–53.
2. Bertrand Y, Landais P, Friedrich W, et al. Influence of severe combined immunodeficiency phenotype on the outcome of HLA non-identical, T-cell-depleted bone marrow transplantation: a retrospective European survey from the European group for bone marrow transplantation and the European society for immunodeficiency. J Pediatr 1999;134(6):740–8.
3. Antoine C, Müller S, Cant A, et al. Long-term survival and transplantation of haemopoietic stem cells for immunodeficiencies: report of the European experience 1968–99. Lancet 2003;361(9357):553–60.
4. Mazzolari E, Forino C, Guerci S, et al. Long-term immune reconstitution and clinical outcome after stem cell transplantation for severe T-cell immunodeficiency. J Allergy Clin Immunol 2007;120(4):892–9.
5. Grunebaum E, Mazzolari E, Porta F, et al. Bone marrow transplantation for severe combined immune deficiency. JAMA 2006;295(5):508–18.
6. Schwarz K, Gauss G, Ludwig L, et al. RAG mutations in human B cell-negative SCID. Science 1996;274(5284):97–9.
7. Noordzij J, Verkaik N, van der Burg M, et al. Radiosensitive SCID patients with Artemis gene mutations show a complete B-cell differentiation arrest at the pre-B-cell receptor checkpoint in bone marrow. Blood 2003;101(4):1446–52.
8. van der Burg M, Ijspeert H, Verkaik N, et al. A DNA-PKcs mutation in a radiosensitive T-B- SCID patient inhibits Artemis activation and nonhomologous end-joining. J Clin Invest 2009;119(1):91–8.
9. Savitsky K, Bar-Shira A, Gilad S, et al. A single ataxia telangiectasia gene with a product similar to PI-3 kinase. Science 1995;268(5218):1749–53.
10. Griffith E, Walker S, Martin C, et al. Mutations in pericentrin cause Seckel syndrome with defective ATR-dependent DNA damage signaling. Nat Genet 2008;40(2):232–6.

11. Gennery A, Slatter M, Bhattacharya A, et al. The clinical and biological overlap between Nijmegen breakage syndrome and Fanconi anemia. Clin Immunol 2004;113(2):214–9.

12. Walker J, Corpina R, Goldberg J. Structure of the Ku heterodimer bound to DNA and its implications for double-strand break repair. Nature 2001;412(6847): 607–14.

13. Ma Y, Pannicke U, Schwarz K, et al. Hairpin opening and overhang processing by an Artemis/DNA-dependent protein kinase complex in non-homologous end joining and V(D)J recombination. Cell 2002;108(6):781–94.

14. Critchlow S, Bowater R, Jackson S. Mammalian DNA double-strand break repair protein XRCC4 interacts with DNA ligase IV. Curr Biol 1997;7(8):588–98.

15. Grawunder U, Wilm M, Wu X, et al. Activity of DNA ligase IV stimulated by complex formation with XRCC4 protein in mammalian cells. Nature 1997; 388(6641):492–5.

16. Ahnesorg P, Smith P, Jackson S. XLF interacts with the XRCC4-DNA ligase IV complex to promote DNA non-homologous end-joining. Cell 2006;124(2): 301–13.

17. Musio A, Marrella V, Sobacchi C, et al. Damaging-agent sensitivity of Artemis-deficient cell lines. Eur J Immunol 2005;35(4):1250–6.

18. Sanderson B, Shield A. Mutagenic damage to mammalian cells by therapeutic alkylating agents. Mutat Res 1996;355(1–2):41–57.

19. O'Driscoll M, Jeggo P. CsA can induce DNA double-strand breaks: implications for BMT regimens particularly for individuals with defective DNA repair. Bone Marrow Transplant 2008;41(11):983–9.

20. Cavazzana-Calvo M, Le Deist F, De Saint Basile G, et al. Increased radiosensitivity of granulocyte macrophage colony-forming units and skin fibroblasts in human autosomal recessive severe combined immunodeficiency. J Clin Invest 1993;91(3):1214–8.

21. Nicolas N, Moshous D, Cavazzana-Calvo M, et al. A human severe combined immunodeficiency (SCID) condition with increased sensitivity to ionizing radiations and impaired V(D)J rearrangements defines a new DNA recombination/repair deficiency. J Exp Med 1998;188(4):627–34.

22. Nicolas N, Finnie NJ, Cavazzana-Calvo M, et al. Lack of detectable defect in DNA double-strand break repair and DNA-dependent protein kinase activity in radiosensitive human severe combined immunodeficiency fibroblasts. Eur J Immunol 1996;26:1118–22.

23. Ege M, Ma Y, Manfras B, et al. Omenn syndrome due to Artemis mutations. Blood 2005;105(11):4179–86.

24. Xiao Z, Yannone S, Dunn E, et al. A novel missense RAG-1 mutation results in T-B-NK+ SCID in Athabascan-speaking Dine Indians from the Canadian Northwest Territories. Eur J Hum Genet 2009;17(2):205–12.

25. Hamby K, Trexler A, Pearson TC, et al. NK cells rapidly reject allogeneic bone marrow in the spleen through a perforin- and Ly49D-dependent, but NKG2D-independent mechanism. Am J Transplant 2007;7(8):1884–96.

26. Murphy WJ, Kumar V, Bennett M. Rejection of bone marrow allografts by mice with severe combined immune deficiency (SCID). Evidence that natural killer cells can mediate the specificity of marrow graft rejection. J Exp Med 1987; 165(4):1212–7.

27. Bailey S, Meyne J, Chen D, et al. DNA double-strand break repair proteins are required to cap the ends of mammalian chromosomes. Proc Natl Acad Sci U S A 1999;96(26):14899–904.

28. Soulas-Sprauel P, Le Guyader G, Rivera-Munoz P, et al. Role for DNA repair factor XRCC4 in immunoglobulin class switch recombination. J Exp Med 2007;204(7): 1717–27.

29. Jones J, Ritenbaugh C, Spence M, et al. Severe combined immunodeficiency among the Navajo. I. Characterization of phenotypes, epidemiology, and population genetics. Hum Biol 1991;63(5):669–82.

30. Moshous D, Li L, Chasseval R, et al. A new gene involved in DNA double-strand break repair and V(D)J recombination is located on human chromosome 10p. Hum Mol Genet 2000;9(4):583–8.

31. Li L, Moshous D, Zhou Y, et al. A founder mutation in Artemis, an SNM1-like protein, causes SCID in Athabascan-speaking Native Americans. J Immunol 2002;168(12):6323–9.

32. Moshous D, Callebaut I, de Chasseval R, et al. Artemis, a novel DNA double-strand break repair/V(D)J recombination protein, is mutated in human severe combined immune deficiency. Cell 2001;105(2):177–86.

33. Kobayashi N, Agematsu K, Sugita K, et al. Novel Artemis gene mutations of radiosensitive severe combined immunodeficiency in Japanese families. Hum Genet 2003;112(4):348–52.

34. O'Marcaigh AS, DeSantes K, Hu D, et al. Bone marrow transplantation for T-B-severe combined immunodeficiency disease in Athabascan-speaking native Americans. Bone Marrow Transplant 2001;27(7):703–9.

35. Friedrich W, Hönig M, Müller S. Long-term follow-up in patients with severe combined immunodeficiency treated by bone marrow transplantation. Immunol Res 2007;38(1–3):165–73.

36. Slatter M, Brigham K, Dickinson A, et al. Long-term immune reconstitution after anti-CD52-treated or anti-CD34-treated hematopoietic stem cell transplantation for severe T-lymphocyte immunodeficiency. J Allergy Clin Immunol 2008;121(2): 361–7.

37. van der Burg M, Weemaes CM, Preijers F, et al. B-cell recovery after stem cell transplantation of Artemis-deficient SCID requires elimination of autologous bone marrow precursor-B-cells. Haematologica 2006;91(12):1705–9.

38. Neven B, Leroy S, Decaluwe H, et al. Long-term outcome after haematopoietic stem cell transplantation of a single-centre cohort of 90 patients with severe combined immunodeficiency: long-term outcome of HSCT in SCID. Blood 2009;113(7):4114–24.

39. Moshous D, Pannetier C, Chasseval RR, et al. Partial T and B lymphocyte immunodeficiency and predisposition to lymphoma in patients with hypomorphic mutations in Artemis. J Clin Invest 2003;111(3):381–7.

40. Frank K, Sekiguchi J, Seidl K, et al. Late embryonic lethality and impaired V(D)J recombination in mice lacking DNA ligase IV. Nature 1998;396(6707):173–7.

41. O'Driscoll M, Cerosaletti K, Girard P, et al. DNA ligase IV mutations identified in patients exhibiting developmental delay and immunodeficiency. Mol Cell 2001; 8(6):1175–85.

42. Buck D, Moshous D, de Chasseval R, et al. Severe combined immunodeficiency and microcephaly in siblings with hypomorphic mutations in DNA ligase IV. Eur J Immunol 2006;36(1):224–35.

43. Enders A, Fisch P, Schwarz K, et al. A severe form of human combined immunodeficiency due to mutations in DNA ligase IV. J Immunol 2006;176(8):5060–8.

44. Nariaki T, Norikazu H, Satoru O, et al. Epstein-Barr virus-associated B-cell lymphoma in a patient with DNA ligase IV (LIG4) syndrome. Am J Med Genet Part A 2007;143(7):742–5.

45. Gruhn B, Seidel J, Zintl F, et al. Successful bone marrow transplantation in a patient with DNA ligase IV deficiency and bone marrow failure. Orphanet J Rare Dis 2007;2:5.
46. Dvorak C, Sandford A, Fong A, et al. Maternal T-cell engraftment associated with severe hemophagocytosis of the bone marrow in untreated X-linked severe combined immunodeficiency. J Pediatr Hematol Oncol 2008;30(5):396–400.
47. van der Burg M, van Veelen L, Verkaik N, et al. A new type of radiosensitive T-B-NK+ severe combined immunodeficiency caused by a LIG4 mutation. J Clin Invest 2006;116(1):137–45.
48. Plowman PN, Bridges BA, Arlett CF, et al. An instance of clinical radiation morbidity and cellular radiosensitivity, not associated with ataxia-telangiectasia. Br J Radiol 1990;63(752):624–8.
49. Riballo E, Critchlow S, Teo S, et al. Identification of a defect in DNA ligase IV in a radiosensitive leukaemia patient. Curr Biol 1999;9(13):699–702.
50. Ben-Omran T, Cerosaletti K, Concannon P, et al. A patient with mutations in DNA Ligase IV: clinical features and overlap with Nijmegen breakage syndrome. Am J Med Genet A 2005;137(3):283–7.
51. Blunt T, Finnie N, Taccioli G, et al. Defective DNA-dependent protein kinase activity is linked to V(D)J recombination and DNA repair defects associated with the murine scid mutation. Cell 1995;80(5):813–23.
52. Wiler R, Leber R, Moore B, et al. Equine severe combined immunodeficiency: a defect in V(D)J recombination and DNA-dependent protein kinase activity. Proc Natl Acad Sci U S A 1995;92(25):11485–9.
53. Meek K, Kienker L, Dallas C, et al. SCID in Jack Russell terriers: a new animal model of DNA-PKcs deficiency. J Immunol 2001;167(4):2142–50.
54. Muller C, Calsou P, Salles B. The activity of the DNA-dependent protein kinase (DNA-PK) complex is determinant in the cellular response to nitrogen mustards. Biochimie 2000;82(1):25–8.
55. Shen H, Schultz M, Kruh G, et al. Increased expression of DNA-dependent protein kinase confers resistance to adriamycin. Biochim Biophys Acta 1998;1381(2):131–8.
56. Jin S, Inoue S, Weaver D. Differential etoposide sensitivity of cells deficient in the Ku and DNA-PKcs components of the DNA-dependent protein kinase. Carcinogenesis 1998;19(6):965–71.
57. Kwong P, O'Marcaigh A, Howard R, et al. Oral and genital ulceration: a unique presentation of immunodeficiency in Athabascan-speaking American Indian children with severe combined immunodeficiency. Arch Dermatol 1999;135(8):927–31.
58. Buck D, Malivert L, de Chasseval R, et al. Cernunnos, a novel nonhomologous end-joining factor, is mutated in human immunodeficiency with microcephaly. Cell 2006;124(2):287–99.
59. Faraci M, Lanino E, Micalizzi C, et al. Unrelated hematopoietic stem cell transplantation for Cernunnos-XLF deficiency. Pediatr Transplant 2009;13(6):785–9.
60. Rubocki RJ, Parsa JR, Hershfield MS, et al. Full hematopoietic engraftment after allogeneic bone marrow transplantation without cytoreduction in a child with severe combined immunodeficiency. Blood 2001;97(3):809–11.
61. Villa A, Notarangelo L, Roifman C. Omenn syndrome: inflammation in leaky severe combined immunodeficiency. J Allergy Clin Immunol 2008;122(6):1082–6.
62. Grunebaum E, Bates A, Roifman CM. Omenn syndrome is associated with mutations in DNA ligase IV. J Allergy Clin Immunol 2008;122(6):1219–20.

63. Muller S, Ege M, Pottharst A, et al. Transplacentally acquired maternal T lymphocytes in severe combined immunodeficiency: a study of 121 patients. Blood 2001;98(6):1847–51.

64. Knobloch C, Goldmann SF, Friedrich W. Limited T cell receptor diversity of transplacentally acquired maternal T cells in severe combined immunodeficiency. J Immunol 1991;146(12):4157–64.

65. Buckley RH, Schiff SE, Schiff RI, et al. Hematopoietic stem-cell transplantation for the treatment of severe combined immunodeficiency. N Engl J Med 1999;340(7): 508–16.

66. Dvorak C, Cowan M. Hematopoietic stem cell transplantation for primary immunodeficiency disease. Bone Marrow Transplant 2008;41(2):119–26.

67. Palmer K, Green TD, Roberts JL, et al. Unusual clinical and immunologic manifestations of transplacentally acquired maternal T cells in severe combined immunodeficiency. J Allergy Clin Immunol 2007;120(2):423–8.

68. Dvorak C, Hung G, Horn B, et al. Megadose CD34(+) cell grafts improve recovery of T cell engraftment but not B cell immunity in patients with severe combined immunodeficiency disease undergoing haplocompatible nonmyeloablative transplantation. Biol Blood Marrow Transplant 2008;14(10):1125–33.

69. Dvorak C, Gilman A, Horn B, et al. Clinical and immunologic outcomes following haplocompatible donor lymphocyte infusions. Bone Marrow Transplant 2009. [Epub ahead of print].

70. Horn B, Bao L, Dunham K, et al. Infusion of cytomegalovirus specific cytotoxic T lymphocytes from a sero-negative donor can facilitate resolution of infection and immune reconstitution. Pediatr Infect Dis J 2009;28(1):65–7.

71. Perruccio K, Tosti A, Burchielli E, et al. Transferring functional immune responses to pathogens after haploidentical hematopoietic transplantation. Blood 2005; 106(13):4397–406.

72. Karlsson H, Brewin J, Kinnon C, et al. Generation of trispecific cytotoxic T cells recognizing cytomegalovirus, adenovirus, and Epstein-Barr virus: an approach for adoptive immunotherapy of multiple pathogens. J Immunother 2007;30(5): 544–56.

73. Kline R, Stiehm E, Cowan M. Bone marrow 'boosts' following T cell-depleted haploidentical bone marrow transplantation. Bone Marrow Transplant 1996;17:543–8.

74. Booth C, Ribeil J, Audat F, et al. CD34 stem cell top-ups without conditioning after initial haematopoietic stem cell transplantation for correction of incomplete haematopoietic and immunological recovery in severe congenital immunodeficiencies. Br J Haematol 2006;135(4):533–7.

75. Cohen A, Békássy A, Gaiero A, et al. Endocrinological late complications after hematopoietic SCT in children. Bone Marrow Transplant 2008;41(Suppl 2):S43–8.

76. Kramer J, Crittenden M, DeSantes K, et al. Cognitive and adaptive behavior 1 and 3 years following bone marrow transplantation. Bone Marrow Transplant 1997;19(6):607–13.

77. Titman P, Pink E, Skucek E, et al. Cognitive and behavioral abnormalities in children after hematopoietic stem cell transplantation for severe congenital immunodeficiencies. Blood 2008;112(9):3907–13.

78. Baker KS, DeFor TE, Burns LJ, et al. New malignancies after blood or marrow stem-cell transplantation in children and adults: incidence and risk factors. J Clin Oncol 2003;21(7):1352–8.

79. Bielorai B, Trakhtenbrot L, Amariglio N, et al. Multilineage hematopoietic engraftment after allogeneic peripheral blood stem cell transplantation without conditioning in SCID patients. Bone Marrow Transplant 2004;34(4):317–20.

80. Bolinger A, Zangwill A, Slattery J, et al. An evaluation of engraftment, toxicity and busulfan concentration in children receiving bone marrow transplantation for leukemia or genetic disease. Bone Marrow Transplant 2000;25(9):925–30.

81. Rao K, Amrolia PJ, Jones A, et al. Improved survival after unrelated donor bone marrow transplantation in children with primary immunodeficiency using a reduced-intensity conditioning regimen. Blood 2005;105(2):879–85.

82. Veys P, Rao K, Amrolia P. Stem cell transplantation for congenital immunodeficiencies using reduced-intensity conditioning. Bone Marrow Transplant 2005; 35(S1):S45–7.

83. Dror Y, Gallagher R, Wara DW, et al. Immune reconstitution in severe combined immunodeficiency disease after lectin-treated, T-cell-depleted haplocompatible bone marrow transplantation. Blood 1993;81(8):2021–30.

84. Mantovani A, Luini W, Peri G, et al. Effect of chemotherapeutic agents on natural cell-mediated cytotoxicity in mice. J Natl Cancer Inst 1978;61(5):1255–61.

85. Robertson L, Denny A, Huh Y, et al. Natural killer cell activity in chronic lymphocytic leukemia patients treated with fludarabine. Cancer Chemother Pharmacol 1996;37(5):445–50.

86. Penack O, Fischer L, Stroux A, et al. Serotherapy with thymoglobulin and alemtuzumab differentially influences frequency and function of natural killer cells after allogeneic stem cell transplantation. Bone Marrow Transplant 2008;41(4):377–83.

87. Rooney S, Sekiguchi J, Zhu C, et al. Leaky Scid phenotype associated with defective V(D)J coding end processing in Artemis-deficient mice. Mol Cell 2002;10(6):1379–90.

88. Xiao Z, Dunn E, Singh K, et al. A non-leaky Artemis-deficient mouse that accurately models the human severe combined immune deficiency phenotype, including resistance to hematopoietic stem cell transplantation. Biol Blood Marrow Transplant 2009;15(1):1–11.

89. Nijnik A, Dawson S, Crockford T, et al. Impaired lymphocyte development and antibody class switching and increased malignancy in a murine model of DNA ligase IV syndrome. J Clin Invest 2009;119(6):1696–705.

90. Li G, Alt F, Cheng H, et al. Lymphocyte-specific compensation for XLF/cernunnos end-joining functions in V(D)J recombination. Mol Cell 2008;31(5):631–40.

91. Chen J, Larochelle A, Fricker S, et al. Mobilization as a preparative regimen for hematopoietic stem cell transplantation. Blood 2006;107(9):3764–71.

92. Czechowicz A, Kraft D, Weissman I, et al. Efficient transplantation via antibody-based clearance of hematopoietic stem cell niches. Science 2007;318(5854): 1296–9.

93. Bhattacharyya S, Chawla A, Smith K, et al. Multilineage engraftment with minimal graft-versus-host disease following in utero transplantation of S-59 psoralen/ultraviolet A light-treated, sensitized T cells and adult T cell-depleted bone marrow in fetal mice. J Immunol 2002;169(11):6133–40.

94. Mostoslavsky G, Fabian A, Rooney S, et al. Complete correction of murine Artemis immunodeficiency by lentiviral vector-mediated gene transfer. Proc Natl Acad Sci U S A 2006;103(44):16406–11.

95. Lagresle-Peyrou C, Benjelloun F, Hue C, et al. Restoration of human B-cell differentiation into NOD-SCID mice engrafted with gene-corrected CD34+ cells isolated from Artemis or RAG1-deficient patients. Mol Ther 2008;16(2):396–403.

Neurocognitive Function of Patients with Severe Combined Immunodeficiency

Ami J. Shah, MD[a],*, Donald B. Kohn, MD[b,c]

KEYWORDS

• SCID • Neurocognitive function • Late effects

In 1968, hematopoietic stem cell transplantation (HSCT) offered the first cure for severe combined immunodeficiency (SCID).[1] Since then, HSCT has been the treatment of choice for patients with SCID. Although HSCT can be curative, there are many long-term complications that can occur. Studies of patients with leukemia after HSCT have shown several long-term complications including neurocognitive delays, endocrinopathies, organ dysfunction, and secondary malignancies. Understanding the neurodevelopmental outcomes in SCID is challenging because multiple factors may influence cognitive and behavioral function. SCID has multiple genetic causes, and the treatments for SCID using HSCT may or may not involve cytoreductive conditioning with chemotherapy before HSCT. It is vital to gain this understanding, to guide treatment approaches, and to provide the optimal psychosocial support to patients with SCID after HSCT.

As the number of survivors after HSCT for SCID increases, there is a growing concern regarding the late effects in this population of patients. Achieving normal developmental milestones after transplant is an integral part of pediatric management. One of the emerging concerns post-HSCT is the neurocognitive function in patients with SCID. The adverse effects associated with neurocognitive function are defined

The authors have no conflicts of interest to declare.

[a] Division of Research Immunology/Bone Marrow Transplantation, Department of Pediatrics, The Saban Research Institute, Childrens Hospital Los Angeles, University of Southern California Keck School of Medicine, 4650 Sunset Boulevard, MS # 62, Los Angeles, CA 90027, USA

[b] Department of Microbiology, Immunology and Molecular Genetics, University of California, Los Angeles, 290D BSRB, 615 Charles E. Young Drive South, Los Angeles, CA 90095, USA

[c] Department of Pediatrics, University of California, Los Angeles, 290D BSRB, 615 Charles E. Young Drive South, Los Angeles, CA 90095, USA

* Corresponding author.

E-mail address: Ashah@chla.usc.edu (A.J. Shah).

as problems that are related to development such as thinking, learning, and memory. Neurodevelopmental outcomes can be assessed by formal, age-appropriate standardized testing, or by functional outcomes, such as school performance.

NEUROCOGNITIVE FUNCTION OF HSCT RECIPIENTS (MALIGNANT AND NONMALIGNANT DISEASES)

Despite the increasing number of survivors of SCID after HSCT, there are limited studies that have been performed on this population. In most studies of neurocognitive function post-HSCT, most patients have had a malignant disease and most patients with nonmalignant disease have not had SCID. Most studies performed on children post-HSCT have combined recipients of HSCT for both malignant and nonmalignant diseases and included patients of different ages, with various diseases, conditioning regimens, and stem cell sources. Previous conditioning regimens in these series of post-HSCT patients consisted of either regimens that included irradiation or those that administered chemotherapy alone without irradiation. But the standard conditioning regimens that have been used for patients with SCID (eg, busulfan/cyclophosphamide) do not include any cranial irradiation. This has made it difficult to extrapolate the findings to the specific risks for infants with SCID, who are treated at a young age, who may have had prior severe infections but have not received previous chemotherapy, in contrast to the patients with malignant disorders who may or may not receive cytoreductive chemotherapy conditioning before HSCT.

There is a considerable body of information on pediatric patients who have received chemotherapy with or without craniospinal irradiation for the treatment of leukemia that did not include HSCT. When craniospinal irradiation was first used to try to prevent localized central nervous system (CNS) relapses in acute leukemia, dosages of 24 Gy of cranial irradiation were typically used. Outcome studies demonstrated that this dosage of radiation to the CNS produced at least an 11-point reduction in global IQ, with even more severe effects in the younger patients.[2] Current regimens to try to prevent localized relapses of leukemia in the neuraxis (CNS prophylaxis) typically use lower dosages of craniospinal radiation (eg, 18 Gy) or use combinations of chemotherapeutic agents delivered intrathecally instead of radiation.

From among the published series on post-HSCT outcomes for pediatrics patients, Kramer and colleagues[3] reported the 1- and 3-year outcomes of 67 patients transplanted for both malignant and nonmalignant diseases. This study showed a significant reduction in IQ scores at 1 year post-HSCT. There were 26 patients who were evaluated at 3 years post-HSCT. These patients had no further reduction in their neurocognitive function. Phipps and colleagues[4] performed a prospective longitudinal study of 102 patients at 1 year post-HSCT and 54 patients at 3 years post-HSCT. The patients in this study had a mixture of malignant and nonmalignant diseases. The conditioning regimens consisted of those receiving irradiation and those receiving chemotherapy alone. There were no differences detected in overall cognitive scores between pre-HSCT patients and post-HSCT patients.[4] A follow-up study from the same group in 2008 evaluated 268 patients until 5 years post-HSCT, 34 of whom had a nonmalignant disease. This study showed minimal decreases in overall neurocognitive function. However, there were subgroups of patients who were at higher risk of neurocognitive declines, such as those who had received irradiation, who had graft-versus-host disease (GVHD), and who had undergone an unrelated donor transplantation.[5] Consistently, however, studies of neurocognitive function have shown that younger age at the time of HSCT was a major factor in an increased risk for long-term neurocognitive deficits, especially among those who received irradiation as part of their therapy. Long-term evaluation of children younger than 3 years with leukemia who underwent HSCT showed that they retained average intelligence but suffered from persistent attention deficits at a median of 12 years post-HSCT.[6]

FACTORS INFLUENCING NEUROCOGNITIVE OUTCOME IN PATIENTS WITH SCID POST-HSCT

For patients with SCID, there are 4 specific areas that can affect the neurocognitive function post-HSCT: (1) disease-specific characteristics, such as the molecular defect, (2) psychosocial factors, such as consanguinity and socioeconomic status, (3) the effect of being a chronically ill child, and (4) transplant-related complications, such as toxicities from chemotherapy conditioning and GVHD.

Disease-Specific Characteristics

A major factor in neurocognitive function post-HSCT is the genetic type of SCID. Some molecular defects have more profound immunologic and nonimmunologic sequelae because of their systemic expression. For example, adenosine deaminase (ADA) deficiency is known to be expressed systemically, and effects on other organ systems are well documented.[7–10] Deficiency of ADA results in accumulation of deoxyadenosine and deoxyadenosine triphosphate (dATP),[11] which affects normal methylation reactions, induces apoptosis in thymic lymphocytes,[12] and inhibits ribonucleotide reductase, which is necessary for normal DNA synthesis.[13,14] Unlike other forms of SCID, ADA-deficient patients have several nonimmunologic abnormalities (eg, skeletal, pulmonary, hepatic), which may reflect the importance of ADA in other organ systems. Patients with ADA deficiency are known to have increased cognitive, behavioral, and neurologic deficits when compared with other forms of SCID.[8–10,15] In patients whose gene defect only affects the immune and hematopoietic systems, no long-term behavioral or cognitive deficits would be expected from the genetic defect alone.

In one study, 3 of 23 ADA-deficient patients suffered from cortical blindness and pyramidal and extrapyramidal motor dysfunction.[16] In a separate study, 2 siblings with ADA deficiency exhibited sensorineural hearing loss.[17] In another study of ADA-deficient patients post-HSCT, 6 of 12 surviving patients suffered severe neurologic abnormalities, including mental retardation, muscular hypertonia, problems with coordination and expressive speech, and sensorineural hearing deficits.[18] Although the authors do not know the precise mechanism for this finding, Hirschhorn and colleagues[16] described an ADA-deficient child with severe motor and pyramidal defects, nystagmus, and global developmental delay whose symptoms improved with enzyme replacement, suggesting that there may be a metabolically induced neurologic defect.

Rogers and colleagues[15] performed formal cognitive, behavioral, and neurodevelopmental studies on 11 patients with ADA deficiency post-HSCT compared with age-matched control patients with other forms of SCID post-HSCT. In the ADA-deficient patients, the standardized IQ score showed an inverse correlation with dATP levels at the time of diagnosis, indicating a significant effect from the genetic type of SCID. Behavioral assessments showed that the ADA-deficient patients functioned in the pathologic range on all areas tested when compared with other patients with SCID. In contrast, in this study there were no differences in cognitive abilities between the ADA-deficient patients and those with other forms of SCID. It should be noted however that both the ADA-deficient group and the non–ADA deficient SCID group scored in the below average range when compared with the normal population. Furthermore, in this study, most of the ADA-deficient patients with SCID did not receive conditioning before transplantation; therefore, the effect of cytotoxic drugs as being the cause of the delays could be dismissed.

Titman and colleagues[19] confirmed that there was a difference among patients whose molecular defect was confined to the immune system (γC, JAK 3, IL-7, Rα, RAG1/2) versus those whose genetic defect was more widely expressed (ADA-SCID). These data support the notion that the underlying genetic defect affects the neurocognitive development, regardless of transplantation. There are, as yet, no published data on the neurologic outcomes in patients with the more recently recognized genetic forms of SCID due to defects in the DNA repair enzymes needed for VDJ (variable-diversity-joining) recombination (Artemis, ligase 4, and DNA-PKc), which may have extraimmunologic effects.

Psychosocial Factors

There are many psychosocial factors that can affect the neurocognitive outcomes of not only patients with SCID but also of any patient. Socioeconomic status is well documented as the most important determinant of cognitive and academic function in all children[20] as well as those who have received HSCT.[5] Among patients with primary immune deficiencies, socioeconomic status was also found to strongly correlate with a lower IQ score.[19]

Because patients with SCID may be the product of consanguineous unions, this may affect the outcomes of these patients regardless of other transplant-related factors. Titman and colleagues[19] undertook a study of all immune-deficient patients who received HSCT and showed that even the unaffected siblings of consanguineous parents had lower IQ scores compared with unaffected children of nonconsanguineous parents. The association of IQ and consanguinity suggests that IQ score is not related only to the transplant experience but rather that other inherited traits affecting IQ score are carried through pedigrees.

Effect of Chronic Illness

The potential effects of the disease, intensive therapy, social isolation, and altered family dynamics in a young child are uncertain and cannot be studied well in this rare disease. Pott-Mees[21] documented the profound psychosocial effects of HSCT on a series of pediatric patients (although none with SCID and their families), despite findings of normal neurodevelopment.

Some patients with SCID are diagnosed at birth, due to a previously affected sibling or relative, and have not developed clinical manifestations of their disease before HSCT. Other patients with SCID present later in infancy with severe life-threatening infections, respiratory failure, malnutrition, and failure to thrive. Many patients with SCID have been hospitalized on numerous occasions before establishing the diagnosis, including a significant number who have undergone ventilatory support for some period. Malnutrition is known to have an impact on growth and development. Malnutrition affects not only the motor development but also the developing mind, regardless of the presence of an underlying disease.

It is well established that younger children undergoing HSCT have poor neurocognitive function post-HSCT for both malignant and nonmalignant diseases.[3,4,6] Because most patients with SCID are diagnosed within the first year of life and are transplanted as soon as possible, they are usually young at the time of transplant and are therefore at greater risk of neurocognitive deficits. However, patients with SCID who are younger than 6 months have more successful outcomes in terms of overall survival after HSCT compared with those older than 6 months.[22,23] Children older than 6 months often have developed symptoms such as respiratory infections before HSCT, which can worsen their overall survival. Titman and colleagues[19] used a cutoff age of 3 years and Lin and colleagues[24] used a cutoff age of 8 months in determining if age was a factor in patients with SCID. Neither of these studies showed a difference in neurocognitive function due to age at time of transplant.

Being a chronically ill child often results in extensive periods of time in the hospital. Even after these patients leave the hospital, they remain immunosuppressed and are therefore kept socially isolated from their age-matched peers. Many of these children do not have healthy older siblings. This social isolation can also result in neurocognitive delays, especially in adaptive function.[24] Titman and colleagues[19] showed that admission to the intensive care unit was associated with a decrease in long-term neurocognitive development.

Transplant-Related Factors

There are many transplant-related factors that can affect the long-term neurocognitive function of patients with SCID, including the pretransplant conditioning regimen, the source of donor cells used for the transplant, and the complications that may occur post-HSCT. Because these factors are often interrelated (eg, the choice of stem cell donor source may influence decisions about pretransplant conditioning and posttransplant complications, such as GVHD), it is difficult to isolate the effects of a single variable.

There are various stem cell sources that are potentially available to patients with SCID, including an HLA-matched sibling, a haploidentical parent, a matched unrelated adult donor, or umbilical cord blood. Potential therapeutic options include a matched sibling transplant with or without conditioning, a T cell–depleted haploidentical transplant with or without conditioning, and a matched unrelated HSCT using stem cells of the bone marrow, cord blood, or peripheral blood. The various treatment options influence the survival, with transplant from a matched sibling leading to an overall survival of approximately 90%[25]; from a T cell–depleted haploidentical donor, to 50% to 78%[25,26]; and from matched unrelated donors, to 65% to 75%.[27]

Patients who undergo a matched sibling transplant often do not receive any pretransplant conditioning and therefore do not have the chemotherapy-related issues from direct neurotoxicity. Patients who undergo matched sibling transplant also have less risk of GVHD than those who receive a matched unrelated transplant or haploidentical transplant. In addition, T-cell reconstitution occurs later in those who receive either a matched unrelated or haploidentical transplant than those who receive a matched sibling donor transplant.[25,26] The lack of T-cell reconstitution increases the risk of infections post-HSCT, which can ultimately prolong hospital days and subsequently affect the neurocognitive outcomes.

NEUROCOGNITIVE FUNCTION OF PATIENTS WITH SCID

The number of neurocognitive studies on patients with SCID alone are minimal. Most studies report clinical observations of their patients in terms of attendance in school, which is a functional outcome that can be measured. Neven and colleagues[28] reported the long-term outcomes of 90 patients who had SCID. Among them, 51 patients did not receive any pretransplant conditioning or received only immunosuppression. The remaining 39 received a busulfan-based conditioning regimen. Among 62 patients who were older than 10 years, 58 (88%) had school performances in the normal range, which was defined as 0 to 2 years of delay in primary or secondary school program. Seven of the surviving patients did not achieve any level of graduation. Three patients required transient psychotherapy and 1 developed schizophrenia as an adult. This study did not evaluate if there was a difference between those receiving no chemotherapy conditioning and those who did receive chemotherapy conditioning. Patel and colleagues reported on the outcomes of 25 children who received a haploidentical HSCT or HLA identical matched donor HSCT with no prior marrow conditioning. Of the 10 survivors who received haploidentical HSCT, 2 were homebound due to severe side effects such as a seizure disorder and bronchiolitis obliterans. Of the 5 survivors of a sibling HSCT, 1 child was homebound due to bronchiolitis obliterans. The remaining children were attending either school or college.[29]

There have been 3 reports in which formal standardized neurocognitive testing was performed for recipients of HSCT for SCID. The first by Rogers and colleagues reported the outcomes of 11 ADA-deficient patients with SCID compared with 11 non–ADA deficient patients with SCID after HSCT. The conclusion of this study was that the adverse cognitive deficits in patients with ADA deficiency were caused by the systemic nature of ADA deficiency instead of the transplant procedure itself, because the ADA-deficient patients did not receive any chemotherapy conditioning. Of note in this study was the relationship between donor engraftment and outcome. Eight of the 11 patients with ADA-deficient SCID did not receive any conditioning and developed mixed donor/recipient marrow chimerism. Of the 3 patients who received conditioning before transplant, only 1 had full donor chimerism. This patient had the best neurocognitive function post-HSCT. This particular patient had also received polyethylene glycol-ADA (PEG-ADA) before HSCT, and there is a possibility that the PEG-ADA before transplant may have corrected or improved some of the non-immunologic manifestations of the disease before HSCT.[15]

Titman and colleagues performed a cross-sectional study on 105 patients with congenital immunodeficiencies (56 of whom had SCID or ADA-SCID) surviving after HSCT. In this study, patients were tested using the age-appropriate Wechsler Intelligence Scales[30–32] at one time point post-HSCT. The average age at assessment was 11 years (3.5–25 years), and average time of assessment post-HSCT was 7 years and 7 months (13 months–25 years). This study showed that the underlying genetic disease, presence of ADA-deficient SCID, and consanguinity were each associated with a worse outcome. Patients who had a more severe clinical course post-HSCT (ie, admission to the intensive care unit) had a worse neurocognitive outcome post-HSCT. Lower socioeconomic status was also associated with poor emotional and behavioral outcomes. In the study population as a whole (SCID and non-SCID), there were 92 children in school. Among them, 27% had a statement of Special Education Needs (compared with 2.5% of the general population).[19]

In this same study, the age at transplantation (<3 years vs >3 years), length of stay in the hospital, and chemotherapy conditioning regimen were not significant risk factors for poorer neurologic outcome. This study also compared all patients with a primary congenital immune deficiency who received no transplant conditioning, reduced intensity conditioning, or fully ablative conditioning regimens. In this study, the IQ score was comparable in all 3 groups, suggesting that there was no effect of the pre-transplant conditioning regimen on neurocognitive function.[19]

Recently, the authors' group performed a prospective study on the neurocognitive function of 16 patients with SCID after HSCT. Sixteen patients were tested pre-HSCT and 1 year post-HSCT using the Bayley Scales of Infant Development[33] and the validated Vineland Adaptive Behavior Scales.[34] Eleven patients were evaluated at 3 years post-HSCT, and 4 patients were evaluated 5 years post-HSCT. Both standardized scaled scores and raw scores were analyzed. All patients received a myeloablative conditioning regimen using busulfan followed by either a haploidentical T cell–depleted transplant, a matched unrelated bone marrow transplant, or cord blood transplant. The authors showed that post-HSCT there were significant decreases in the mental development and psychomotor development scores. Although there was a decrease in the scaled scores, the increase in raw scores over time indicated that these children progressively acquired developmental milestones but at a slower rate than normal infants and toddlers. Because many of these children were in the hospital for prolonged periods of time and were socially isolated from other children after they left the hospital, it was felt that the social isolation resulted in some of the adaptive behavioral delays that are seen early post-HSCT. The patients who were available for testing at 5 years post-HSCT had overall development scores that were comparable to their pre-HSCT scores. There was no effect due to the patients' age at the time of HSCT (<8 months vs >8 months), the presence of serious infections pre-HSCT, or the length of stay in the hospital.[24]

PROPOSED LONG-TERM FOLLOW-UP

Given the improved survival post-HSCT for patients with SCID, a prospective plan for follow-up is suggested to detect the neurocognitive deficiencies for which they are at high risk. At the minimum, a full battery of age-appropriate neurocognitive tests should be done after transplantation and continued assessments of these patients should continue every year through the age of 5 years. Once in school, these patients should be evaluated at least every 2 years until they are at least 10 years post-HSCT. Comprehensive ongoing surveillance may be reduced after this point unless there are parental reports of problems. There are many patients who are at significant risk post-HSCT including those with lower socioeconomic status and those with specific genetic defects such as ADA deficiency, who may benefit from ongoing evaluations. Many of these children will need individualized educational plans while in school, and clinicians should remain involved with these children and their families to provide guidance. These children should also be monitored long term to assess for difficulties in behavior, socialization, and schooling.

Finally, the previously published data on outcomes post-HSCT for SCID remain sparse. More collaborative multicenter studies need to be undertaken to compile data to assess not only the neurocognitive function of these patients but also the effect of HSCT on other organ systems and on the quality of life. Large multicenter trials may be able to determine the true effect of specific genetic mutations, conditioning regimens, source of stem cells, infectious complications, and donor chimerism on the long-term outcomes of this rare disease.

REFERENCES

1. Gatti RA, Meuwissen HJ, Allen HD, et al. Immunological reconstitution of sex-linked lymphopenic immunological deficiency. Lancet 1968;2:1366–9.
2. Cousens P, Waters B, Said J, et al. Cognitive effects of cranial irradiation in leukemia therapy: a survey and meta-analysis. J Child Psychol Psychiatry 1988;29:839–52.
3. Kramer JH, Crittendon MR, DeSantes K, et al. Cognitive and adaptive behavior 1and 3 years following bone marrow transplantation. Bone Marrow Transplant 1997;19:607–13.
4. Phipps S, Dunavant M, Srivastava DK, et al. Cognitive and academic functioning in survivors of pediatric bone marrow transplantation. J Clin Oncol 2000;18: 1004–11.
5. Phipps S, Rai SN, Leung WH, et al. Cognitive and academic consequences of stem-cell transplantation in children. J Clin Oncol 2008;26:2027–33.

6. Perkins JL, Kunin-Batson AS, Youngren NM, et al. Long-term follow up of children who underwent hematopoietic cell transplant (HCT) for AML or ALL at less than 3 years of age. Pediatr Blood Cancer 2007;49:958–63.
7. Albuquerque W, Gaspar HB. Bilateral sensorineural deafness in adenosine deaminase deficient severe combined immunodeficiency. J Pediatr 2004;144: 278–80.
8. Bollinger ME, Arredondo-Vega FX, Santiseben I, et al. Brief report: hepatic dysfunction as a somplication of adenosine deaminase defiency. N Engl J Med 1996;334:1367–71.
9. Ratech H, Greco MA, Gallo G, et al. Patholoic findings in adenosine deaminase-deficient severe combined immunodeficiency. I Kidney, adrenal, and chondro-osseous tissue alterations. Am J Pathol 1985;120:157–69.
10. Cedarbaum SD, Kaitila I, Rimoin DL, et al. The chondro-osseous dysplasia of adenosine deaminase deficiency with severe immunodeficiency. J Pediatr 1976;89:737–42.
11. Hirschorn R. Overview of biochemical abnormalities and molecular genetics of adenosine deaminase deficiency. Pediatr Res 1993;33:S35–41.
12. Benveniste P, Cohen A. A p53 expression is required for thymocyte apoptosis induced induced by adenosine deaminase deficiency. Proc Natl Acad Sci U S A 1995;92:8373–7.
13. Takeda E, Kuroda Y, Naito E, et al. Effects of deoxyadenosine on ribonucleotide reductase in adenosine deaminase-deficient lymphocytes. J Inherit Metab Dis 1991;14:87–95.
14. Lee N, Russell N, Ganeshaguru K, et al. Mechanisms of deoxyadenosine toxicity in human lymphoid cells in vitro: relevance to the therapeutic use of inhibitors of adenosine deaminase. Br J Haematol 1984;56:107–19.
15. Rogers MH, Lwin R, Fairbanks L, et al. Cognitive and behavioral abnormalities in adenosine deaminase deficient severe combined immunodeficiency. J Pediatr 2001;139:44–50.
16. Hirschhorn R, Paagerogiou PS, Kessarwala HH, et al. Amelioration of neurologic abnormalities after "enzyme replacement" in adenosine deaminase deficiency. N Engl J Med 1980;303:377–80.
17. Tanaka C, Hara T, Suzaki I, et al. Sensorineural deafness in siblings with adenosine deaminase deficiency. Brain Dev 1996;18:304–6.
18. Hönig M, Albert MH, Schulz A, et al. Patients with adenosine deaminase deficiency surviving after hematopoietic stem cell transplantation are at high risk of CNS complications. Blood 2007;109:3595–602.
19. Titman P, Pink E, Skucek E, et al. Cognitive and behavioral abnormalities in children after hematopoietic stem cell transplantation for severe congenital immunodeficiencies. Blood 2008;112:3907–13.
20. Bradley RH, Corwyn RF. Socioeconomic status and child development. Annu Rev Psychol 2002;53:371–99.
21. Pott-Mees CC. The psychological aspects of bone marrow transplantation in children. Delft (The Netherlands): Eburon; 1989.
22. Dror Y, Gallagher R, Wara DW, et al. Immune reconstitution in severe combined immunodeficiency disease after lectin-treated, T cell depleted haploidentical donors. Eur J Pediatr 1985;81:2021–30.
23. Bertrand Y, Landais P, Friedrich W, et al. Influence of SCID phenotype on the outcome of HLA non-identical T-cell-depleted bone marrow transplantation: a retrospective European group for BMT (EBMT) and the European Society for Immunodeficiency (ESID). J Pediatr 1999;134:740–8.

24. Lin M, Epport K, Azen C, et al. Long-term neurocognitive function of pediatric patients with severe combined immune deficiency (SCID): pre- and post-hematopoietic stem cell transplant (HSCT). J Clin Immunol 2009;29:231–7.
25. Antoine C, Muller S, Cant A, et al. Long term survival and transplantation of haematopoietic stem cells for immunodeficiencies: report of the European experience 1868–99. Lancet 2003;361:553–60.
26. Buckley RH, Schiff SE, Schiff RI, et al. Hematopoietic stem cell transplantation for the treatment of severe combined immunodeficiency. N Engl J Med 1999;340: 508–16.
27. Grunebaum E, Mazzolari E, Porta F, et al. Bone marrow transplantation for severe combined immunodeficiency. JAMA 2006;295:508–18.
28. Neven B, Leroy S, Decaluwe H, et al. Long-term outcome after hematopoietic stem cell transplantation of a single center cohort of 90 patients with severe combined immunodeficiency. Blood 2009;113:4114–24.
29. Patel NC, Chinen J, Rosenblatt HM, et al. Long-term outcomes of nonconditioned patients with severe combined immunodeficiency transplanted with HLA-identical or haploidentical bone marrow depleted of T cells with anti-CD6 mAb. J Allergy Clin Immunol 2008;122:1185–93.
30. Wechsler D. The Wechsler Preschool and Primary Scale of intelligence. 3rd edition. San Antonio (TX): The Psychological Corporation; 2004.
31. Wechsler D. Wechsler Intelligence Scale for children. 3rd edition. San Antonio (TX): The Psychological Corporation; 1992.
32. Wechsler D. Wechsler Adult Intelligence Scale. 3rd edition. San Antonio (TX): The Psychological Corporation; 1999.
33. Bayley N. Bayley Scales of Infant Development. 2nd edition. San Antonio (TX): The Psychological Corporation; 1993.
34. Sparrow SS, Balla DA, Cicchetti DV. Vineland Adaptive Behavior Scales. Circles Pines (MN): American Guidance Service; 1984.

Index

Note: Page numbers of article titles are in **boldface** type.

A

Adenosine deaminase deficiency, stem cell transplantation for, 21–22
    haploidentical and T-cell depleted, 51
    HLA-haploidentical, 40
    neurocognitive function and, 145–146
Alefacept, for graft-versus-host disease, 85
Alemtuzumab, for T-cell depletion, 48
Allogeneic-related stem cell transplantation, for SCID, 18–19
Ancillary Therapy and Supportive Care Working Group, for graft-versus-host disease, 91
Antigen-presenting cells, activation of, in graft-versus-host disease, 78–79
Antithymocyte globulin, for reduced intensity stem cell transplantation, 105, 113
Artemis deficiency, 128–129
Asia-Pacific Blood Marrow Transplant group report, 9

B

B cells, recovery of, after stem cell transplantation, 55
Beclomethasone, for graft-versus-host disease, 83
Bone marrow transplantation. *See* Hematopoietic stem cell transplantation.
Budesonide, for graft-versus-host disease, 83
Busulfan, for stem cell transplantation, 36, 113

C

CD34 cells
    megadose of, after stem cell transplantation, 55–56
    positive selection of, for T-cell depletion, 48
CD52, antibodies to, for T-cell depletion, 48
Cellular effectors, in graft-versus-host disease, 80–81
Center for International Blood and Marrow Transplant Research report, 9
Cernunnos-XLF deficiency, 131–132
Chemokines, in graft-versus-host disease, 80–81
Chimerism
    in primary immunodeficiency disease, 111–112
    in SCID, 27
Chronic granulomatous disease, 107, 119–120
Conditioning, for stem cell transplantation
    from HLA-haploidentical donors, 32–34, 36
    in radiosensitive immunodeficiencies, 134–135
Corticosteroids, for graft-versus-host disease, 83, 87
Cyclophosphamide, for stem cell transplantation
    fludarabine and low-dose total body irradiation with, 114

Immunol Allergy Clin N Am 30 (2010) 153–158
doi:10.1016/S0889-8561(10)00009-3
0889-8561/10/$ – see front matter © 2010 Elsevier Inc. All rights reserved.

immunology.theclinics.com

Moving?

Make sure your subscription moves with you!

To notify us of your new address, find your **Clinics Account Number** (located on your mailing label above your name), and contact customer service at:

Email: journalscustomerservice-usa@elsevier.com

800-654-2452 (subscribers in the U.S. & Canada)
314-447-8871 (subscribers outside of the U.S. & Canada)

Fax number: 314-447-8029

Elsevier Health Sciences Division
Subscription Customer Service
3251 Riverport Lane
Maryland Heights, MO 63043

*To ensure uninterrupted delivery of your subscription, please notify us at least 4 weeks in advance of move.